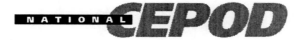

ROYAL COLLEGE OF ANAESTHETISTS

✦

ROYAL COLLEGE OF OBSTETRICIANS AND GYNAECOLOGISTS

✦

ROYAL COLLEGE OF OPHTHALMOLOGISTS

✦

ROYAL COLLEGE OF PATHOLOGISTS

✦

ROYAL COLLEGE OF PHYSICIANS OF LONDON

✦

ROYAL COLLEGE OF RADIOLOGISTS

✦

ROYAL COLLEGE OF SURGEONS OF ENGLAND

✦

FACULTY OF DENTAL SURGERY OF THE ROYAL COLLEGE OF SURGEONS
OF ENGLAND

✦

FACULTY OF PUBLIC HEALTH MEDICINE OF THE ROYAL COLLEGES OF
PHYSICIANS OF THE UK

✦

ASSOCIATION OF ANAESTHETISTS OF GREAT BRITAIN & IRELAND

✦

ASSOCIATION OF SURGEONS OF GREAT BRITAIN & IRELAND

WHO OPERATES WHEN?

A report by the
National Confidential Enquiry into
Perioperative Deaths

(1 April 1995 to 31 March 1996)

E A Campling   BA MHSM DipHSM MBA
H B Devlin   CBE MD FRCS
R W Hoile   MS FRCS
G S Ingram   MBBS FRCA
J N Lunn   MD FRCA

1

Published 30 September 1997

by the National Confidential Enquiry into Perioperative Deaths

35-43 Lincoln's Inn Fields
London
WC2A 3PN

Tel: 0171 831 6430

Requests for further information should be addressed to the Chief Executive

ISBN 0 9522069 4 3

The National Confidential Enquiry into Perioperative Deaths is a company limited by guarantee. Company number 3019382

Contents

Deaths during 1995/96

Appendices

A   Participating hospitals and local contacts
B   The questionnaire
C   Notes about completion of the questionnaire
D   Definitions (NHS Data Dictionary)
E   Tables E1 to E3
    List of procedures performed   18.00 to 21.00 hrs
                                                       21.01 to 24.00 hrs
                                                       00.01 to 07.59 hrs

F   All deaths reported by local reporters
    1 April 1995 to 31 March 1996

Foreword

Previous NCEPOD studies had found that a disturbing number of those who died had undergone their surgery out of hours. There were suspicions that some of these operations were done not because of the urgency of the condition but from want of time in scheduled operating lists, and that patients might be being anaesthetised and operated on by trainee anaesthetists and surgeons working without supervision, but from the data available to it NCEPOD could not relate information derived from postoperative deaths to the overall usage of operating theatres.

The present study was undertaken to define the pattern of surgical activity during a randomised series of 24-hour periods which added up to one week's work for each participating hospital during 1995/96, which would place out-of-hours activity in perspective.

The gathering and handling of such a very large amount of information, involving more than 50,000 cases, posed an unprecedented burden for the staff of NCEPOD, whose willing efforts deserve our thanks and praise; as do those of the many consultants and administrative staff in the participating hospitals, and our advisors, without whose enthusiastic cooperation there could have been no study.

The significant finding was how few (6.1% only) of weekday operations in the NHS were done out of hours, and most of them before midnight. But although they were done out of hours, 93.4% of these were emergencies and indeed most (56%) emergencies arising on a weekday were dealt with during working hours. The reasons given why any were done out of hours, do however give rise to concern: they include lack of daytime theatre facilities; insistence by the anaesthetist on a period of up to six hours preoperative starvation even though a rapid sequence induction would be required; the low priority assigned to operations such as the evacuation of retained products of conception, fractured neck of femur in elderly people and acute appendicitis. These matters have important clinical and educational implications upon which expert independent comments have been obtained for this report.

When, for whatever reason, weekday operations were postponed until out of hours, then many of them were carried out by trainee anaesthetists and surgeons apparently without direct supervision. It should be emphasised that the period of the survey (1995/96) was before the implementation of the Calman report, at a time when many senior house officers and registrars, especially those from overseas, may well have been more experienced than their status might suggest; nevertheless they were in training posts, where unsupervised practice is agreed to have little educational value.

It might be useful to repeat this study in five years' time to see whether there have been changes as a result of the Calman reforms, the introduction of shorter working hours for junior doctors and the promised increase in numbers of consultants.

J P Blandy CBE FRCS
Chairman
National Confidential Enquiry into Perioperative Deaths

V R Tindall CBE MD FRCS FRCOG
Vice-Chairman
National Confidential Enquiry into Perioperative Deaths

September 1997

Summary of findings in NHS hospitals

1   54% (24756/45806) of all operations during the daytime on a weekday were performed in the presence of a consultant surgeon (table 36) and 56% (22286/39767) in the presence of a consultant anaesthetist (table 39).

2   71% (32489/45806) of the operations during the daytime on a weekday were performed in the presence of a trained surgeon, where 'trained surgeon' includes staff grade, associate specialist, senior registrar and consultant (table 36). The figure for 'trained anaesthetists', similarly defined, was 72% (28584/39767, table 39).

3   7% (3221/45806) of the operations during the daytime on a weekday and 20% (509/2550) during weekday evenings were performed by apparently unsupervised senior house officers (tables 36 and 41). The related figures for SHO anaesthetists were 9% (3548/39767, table 39) and 47% (1150/2436, table 43).

4   37% (1309/3531) of the emergency procedures during weekday daytimes (08.00 to 18.00 hrs), and 6.3% (148/2346) during weekday evenings (18.01 to 24.00 hrs) were performed during sessions scheduled primarily for emergency theatre cases (tables 16 and 18). The overall percentage (08.00 to 24.00 hrs) was 25% (1457/5877).

5   51% (182/355) of the participating hospitals had scheduled operating sessions for emergency procedures during the day from Monday to Friday (page 28).

6   46% (19299/42320) of the routine cases started during the daytime from Monday to Friday were day cases (table 25).

7   The imbalance between 'trained' and 'untrained' medical staff is even more apparent at night and at weekends (tables 45 and 48, 50 and 51 respectively).

Recommendations

1 All hospitals admitting emergency surgical patients must be of sufficient size to provide 24-hour operating rooms and other critical care services. There should also be sufficient medical staff to perform these functions.

2 These provisions should be continuous throughout the year: trauma and acute surgical emergencies do not recognise weekends or public holidays.

3 Patients now expect to be treated and managed by trained and competent staff. Patients assume trainees to be taught appropriately and supervised as necessary. Consultants should acknowledge these facts and react accordingly.

Implementation

Organisational

- All hospitals which admit patients for emergency procedures should have an emergency surgery list, staffed and in a fully-equipped theatre suite. Anaesthetists and surgeons rostered for emergency work should be free from other commitments: this should be a fixed part of the consultant contract.

- Consultant anaesthetists, surgeons and hospital managers should *together* plan the administration and management of emergency admissions and procedures.

- In order to avoid queuing for theatre space it may be necessary to nominate an *arbitrator* in theatres who would decide the relative priority of theatre cases. This practice already successfully operates in some hospitals and should be used more widely.

- All hospitals should record the grades of anaesthetists and surgeons present in the anaesthetic room and the operating theatre and their responsibilities.

- Systematic clinical audit should include the pattern of work in the operating theatres.

- An attempt to harmonise the definitions used by the NHS Executive, and the clinical definitions commonly used by surgeons and anaesthetists, would be welcome.

Clinical

- The condition of patients should be optimised prior to anaesthesia and surgery. This may involve the use of local protocols addressing issues such as: the required duration of preoperative starvation, the use of emergency admission units/wards, the preoperative use of critical care services (ICU/HDU etc.), the management of comorbidities by other consultant medical specialists as appropriate, fluid management, analgesia and appropriate use of facilities for the elderly.

Summary of the method

Between 1 April 1995 and 31 March 1996, data were provided to NCEPOD from 355 hospitals in the NHS and 22 independent sector hospitals about surgical procedures performed over seven 24-hour periods. The dates for the data collection were specified by NCEPOD and each of the seven dates for a Trust or unit occurred on a different day of the week.

NCEPOD defined as "out-of-hours" any surgical procedure for which the start of anaesthesia, or the start of the procedure, was between 18.01 and midnight (evening), or midnight and 07.59 hours (night-time), or the procedure was performed on a Saturday, Sunday or bank holiday. For these out-of-hours cases, the consultant surgeon or gynaecologist was asked to confirm or amend the starting time and other details and to state why the procedure was performed at that time.

The local contacts who had provided the initial data were asked also to inform NCEPOD of the death of any patient whose procedure was performed on the days studied. These were restricted to deaths within 30 days of that procedure. The relevant consultant surgeon and anaesthetist were asked to complete questionnaires about these patients.

Setting up the study

The first stage in planning the study was to devise a draft questionnaire for collection of the initial data on all surgical procedures and to ascertain whether all of the data could be provided by the participating hospitals. In December 1994, a draft questionnaire was sent to the Chief Executive of the relevant NHS Trusts or units in England, Wales and Northern Ireland. The NCEPOD administrative team had already identified the NHS hospitals in which surgical procedures were performed. The draft questionnaire was also sent to the manager of Benenden Hospital and hospitals managed by BUPA Hospitals Ltd, Compass Healthcare, BMI Healthcare, Nuffield Hospitals and St Martins Hospitals Limited.

Participation (NHS)

The Chief Executives of 220 NHS Trusts agreed to provide the data via a named contact person within the Trust. The participating Trusts and hospitals are listed in Appendix A; the regional spread of the hospitals is shown below.

Number of hospitals in the study

	Hospitals	Trusts
Anglia and Oxford	23	17
North Thames	48	31
North West	53	32
Northern and Yorkshire	39	23
South Thames	46	25
South & West	38	19
Trent	23	19
West Midlands	41	23
Northern Ireland	20	13
Wales	24	18
Total	**355**	**220**

The lack of a computerised theatre information system (or missing links with other systems) in some hospitals precluded participation in the study; Chief Executives commented that the workload of collecting the data manually would be too great. However, many of the participating hospitals provided the data without the aid of a computerised system, and this represented many hours of clerical or clinical time. In two Trusts, work on other clinical audit projects (internal and external) in the operating theatres prevented participation in the NCEPOD study.

Participation (independent sector)

BUPA	18
BMI Healthcare	3
Benenden Hospital	1

The response from the independent sector was disappointing. The managers of 18 BUPA hospitals agreed to participate, but the remaining 11 were unable to do so. Only two of the BMI Healthcare managers were able to join the study although another four had originally indicated their willingness to provide data. Nuffield Hospitals and St Martins Hospitals each made a corporate decision not to participate. These independent hospital groups were advised by the Independent Healthcare Association not to participate.

The questionnaire and method

Chief Executives provided helpful comments on the proposed methodology and draft questionnaire, which was designed to collect data on every surgical procedure performed in each hospital over seven 24-hour periods between 1 April 1995 and 31 March 1996. Amendments were made to the questionnaire, reproduced as Appendix B.

The main change to the method was to agree that NCEPOD would specify the data collection dates two weeks in advance, rather than retrospectively, on the understanding that the local contact would restrict knowledge of this date to those responsible for data collection. Many of the Chief Executives stated that some of the data required were not routinely recorded and would need to be collected specifically for the NCEPOD study.

The method for this study was therefore finalised as described below.

- Chief Executives of all participating hospitals to identify a person who will provide the initial data to NCEPOD.

- NCEPOD to contact people who will provide data.

- From 1 April 1995, the initial questionnaire should be completed for all surgical procedures performed during a 24-hour period specified by NCEPOD.

- Each hospital will provide data on seven days throughout the year. These days will fall in different weeks.

- NCEPOD will inform the contact of the relevant day two weeks in advance of each date.

- If the contact is unavailable (e.g. on annual leave) an alternative date will be selected.

- All data from the completed questionnaires as received will be entered to the NCEPOD database

- For all "out-of-hours" surgery (evening and night-time on weekdays, plus weekends and bank holidays) a letter will be sent to the Consultant Surgeon to ask for further information on why the operation was performed at this time.

- The local contact will be asked to inform NCEPOD of any patients included in the initial data collection who die within 30 days of this procedure.

- Detailed questionnaires will be sent about these patients who have died, to the Consultant Surgeon and Consultant Anaesthetist.

A local coordinator was identified for each hospital and an information pack about the study was sent to each of them. The pack included notes about completion of the questionnaire (Appendix C) and definitions of terms used (Appendix D).

We are indebted to the local coordinators and to all of the people who collected data. We have named as many as possible of these people individually in Appendix A. The study would have been impossible without their hard work and enthusiasm.

Running the study

Confidentiality

The study was conducted under strict rules of confidentiality, according to the overall NCEPOD protocol and the Enquiry's registration with the Data Protection Registrar.

Allocation of dates

A code number was allocated to each participating Trust. Seven dates were allocated to each hospital on a random basis, ensuring that each of the seven dates fell on a different day of the week. The local contact was informed by letter two weeks in advance of the date and was asked to liaise with a specific member of the NCEPOD staff about any problems. Copies of the questionnaire were then sent from the NCEPOD office in time for the data collection date.

Recording the data

The forms were returned to NCEPOD with a cover sheet on which comments could be made about any difficulties or unusual circumstances of the data. All data from these questionnaires were entered onto the NCEPOD database. NCEPOD staff liaised with the local contacts about omissions or queries in the data. A total of 53162 questionnaires (each one referring to one procedure only) were included, after exclusion of inappropriate questionnaires.

The surgical procedures were all coded using the "Classification of Surgical Operations and Procedures, fourth revision" of the Office of Population Censuses and Surveys.

Deaths

Approximately one month after the operation date or receipt of the completed questionnaires, we requested details of any patients who had died within 30 days of the procedure. A summary of the data originally provided by the local contact accompanied this request. When a death was reported, a detailed questionnaire was sent to the consultant surgeon and consultant anaesthetist involved. These were similar to those used in previous NCEPOD studies (refs) and copies are available on request from the NCEPOD office. First and second reminder letters were sent when necessary. Data from these questionnaires were entered onto the NCEPOD database.

Out-of-hours cases

All of the procedures performed between 18.01 hrs and midnight, and between midnight and 07.59 hrs on weekdays, or at any time on a Saturday, Sunday or public holiday were designated as "out-of-hours" by NCEPOD. The consultant surgeon was asked to validate the information about the procedure, the grade of the operating surgeon and the starting time for each of the procedures. The short questionnaire sent to the consultant surgeon also requested information about the reasons for the timing of the procedure. The replies were coded and entered onto the database.

Data analysis and review

Aggregated data

The data were analysed by the Chief Executive. Aggregated data were provided to the NCEPOD Steering Group, clinical coordinators and advisors within the strict rules of confidentiality of NCEPOD. Individual Trusts, hospitals and clinicians were not identified.

Selection of advisors

In April 1996, postgraduate medical deans were each asked to nominate:

- one specialist registrar within his or her final year of training in anaesthesia
- two specialist registrars within their final year of training in surgery (any specialty) or gynaecology
- two consultant surgeons or gynaecologists

Regional specialty advisors (of The Royal College of Surgeons of England) were also each asked to nominate one specialist registrar and one consultant surgeon in the relevant specialty.

The NCEPOD clinical coordinators selected advisors from these nominations, aiming to achieve even representation across the English regions, Wales and Northern Ireland.

Advisory groups

NCEPOD is extremely grateful to the anaesthetists, gynaecologists and surgeons who attended meetings and who provided valuable advice and commentary on the data. They are listed on page 15.

Review of the data and questionnaires

The advisors reviewed aggregated data on the surgical procedures and the deaths. All replies from consultant surgeons about the reasons for out-of-hours operating were also reviewed. These sheets were rendered anonymous by the NCEPOD administrative staff so that the source of the information was not identifiable.

In addition, questionnaires about the small number of deaths were reviewed in detail by the advisory groups.

Specialist registrars in anaesthesia

Dr P Foster	North West
Dr G Greenslade	South West
Dr K Kiff	North Thames
Dr F Mackay	Wales
Dr E de-Melo	Trent
Dr A Pittard	Northern & Yorkshire
Dr J Wace	South & West

Specialist registrars in surgery

Cardiothoracic surgery	Mr J Carey	Northern & Yorkshire
General surgery	Mr I Bailey	South & West
	Miss B Lovett	North Thames
	Mr A Patel	Anglia & Oxford
Gynaecology	Mr J Armatage	North West
	Mr R Naik	Northern & Yorkshire
Orthopaedic surgery	Mr N Giles	Wales
	Mr F Haddad	North Thames
	Mr P J Owen	South Thames
Otorhinolaryngology	Mr G McBride	Northern Ireland
Paediatric surgery	Miss L Huskisson	West Midlands
Plastic surgery	Mr O G Titley	West Midlands
Urology	Mr M Palmer	North West

Mr A Sofat (neurosurgery, South Thames) was also selected but was unable to attend the meetings.

Consultant gynaecologists and surgeons

Cardiothoracic surgery	Mr A Bryan	South & West
General surgery	Mr N Fieldman	North Thames
	Mr I Hutchinson	Northern & Yorkshire
	Mr K D Vellacott	Wales
Gynaecology	Mr J Lane	West Midlands
	Mr J Tidy	Trent
Neurosurgery	Mr T Pigott	North West
Orthopaedic surgery	Mr A Floyd	Anglia & Oxford
	Mr P Laing	Wales
	Mr D McBride	West Midlands
Otorhinolaryngology	Mr J Topham	South Thames
Paediatric surgery	Miss V Wright	North Thames
Plastic surgery	Mrs S A Pape	Northern & Yorkshire
Urology	Mr G Harrison	South & West

The results

The results

Table 1
Number of days in each month for which data were provided

	Monday	Tuesday	Wednesday	Thursday	Friday	Saturday	Sunday	Total
April (1995)	4	4	4	4	4	5	5	30
May	5	5	5	4	4	4	4	31
June	4	4	4	5	5	4	4	30
July	5	4	4	4	4	5	5	31
August	4	5	5	5	4	4	4	31
September	4	4	4	4	5	5	3	29
October	4	5	4	4	4	4	5	30
November	4	4	5	5	4	4	4	30
December	4	4	4	4	5	5	5	31
January	5	5	5	4	4	4	4	31
February	4	4	4	5	4	4	4	29
March (1996)	4	4	4	4	5	5	5	31
Total	51	52	52	52	52	53	52	364

Data were not received for one day in September and one day in October. The total number of days is therefore 364, not 366 (1996 was a leap year).

Table 2
Number of theatre cases

	Monday	Tuesday	Wednesday	Thursday	Friday	Saturday	Sunday	Total
April	333	377	358	728	468	85	78	2427
May	656	1082	866	776	906	155	86	4527
June	684	462	1006	833	987	141	83	4196
July	899	779	550	877	516	181	130	3932
August	553	1140	757	1248	568	115	68	4449
September	803	1129	1209	1046	1159	160	72	5578
October	1086	1001	1076	836	719	201	42	4961
November	1160	992	1064	609	786	141	112	4864
December	756	750	850	923	700	148	127	4254
January	1226	1040	1051	993	693	134	78	5215
February	686	1075	902	937	786	130	114	4630
March	897	578	661	583	1089	236	85	4129
Total	9739	10405	10350	10389	9377	1827	1075	53162

Public holidays are included in all of the tables above. For England and Wales, these were Friday 14 April 1995, Monday 17 April 1995, Monday 8 May 1995, Monday 29 May 1995, Monday 28 August 1995, Monday 25 and Tuesday 26 December 1995 and Monday 1 January 1996. (In Northern Ireland, 12 July 1995 and 17 March 1996 were also public holidays, but no data were requested from Northern Ireland for these dates).

The total of 53162 cases therefore represents very approximately one fiftieth of the annual surgical workload of the participating hospitals during this period.

Independent hospitals

Independent hospitals

The data on 1497 procedures in 22 independent hospitals are included in tables 3, 4.and 5. For the remainder of this report, the data are reviewed separately.

Table 3 (independent hospitals)
Number of individual hospitals/number of theatre cases

	Monday	Tuesday	Wednesday	Thursday	Friday	Saturday	Sunday	Total cases
April	4/45	3/63	2/23	-	-	-	-	131
May	2/37	1/7	4/61	2/30	-	2/21	-	156
June	1/7	3/18	4/63	1/16	3/34	3/15	1/1	154
July	2/27	2/20	2/26	2/25	2/24	1/13	-	135
August	2/29	1/22	1/15	2/22	4/33	1/2	-	123
September	1/8	1/13	3/32	1/8	2/31	-	-	92
October	2/20	2/28	-	2/23	3/39	1/3	-	113
November	2/16	-	-	8/110	1/10	1/2	-	138
December	1/33	2/24	2/10	1/30	2/6	2/7	2/5	115
January	-	3/34	-	-	-	1/9	-	43
February	-	1/9	1/17	1/10	1/14	4/29	-	79
March	2/61	1/20	3/38	1/9	2/25	4/55	1/10	218
Total cases	**283**	**258**	**285**	**283**	**216**	**156**	**16**	**1497**

Table 4 (independent hospitals)
Surgical specialty of the consultant surgeon in charge

	Number of cases	%
General	385	25.7
Gynaecology	293	19.6
Orthopaedic and trauma	270	18.0
Otorhinolaryngology	185	12.4
Urology	110	7.4
Ophthalmic	100	6.7
Oral/maxillofacial	77	5.1
Plastic	42	2.8
Cardiothoracic	20	1.3
Neurosurgery	12	0.8
Paediatric	3	0.2
Total	**1497**	**100**

Consultant surgeons performed 1451 of the procedures; the remaining 46 cases were from two hospitals. Consultant anaesthetists were present for at least 1244 of the 1283 procedures performed in the presence of an anaesthetist (the grade was not known in 16 cases). The non-consultants were working in the two hospitals already mentioned.

Table 5 (independent hospitals)
Starting time of procedures

	Monday to Friday	Saturday	Sunday
00.01 to 07.59	11	-	-
08.00 to 18.00	1200	153	15
18.01 to 22.00	113	3	3
22.01 to 24.00	1	-	-

All of the procedures before 08.00 hrs were started between 07.00 and 07.55 hrs. Only 18 of the cases between 18.01 and 22.00 hrs were started after 20.00 hrs.

NHS hospitals

(Summary data)

NHS hospitals

The remainder of the tables refer to NHS hospitals only.

Summary data (all times)

Table 6
Number of theatre cases (by specialty of the consultant surgeon in charge)

	Monday to Friday❖	%*	Saturday	%*	Sunday	%*	Total
Cardiothoracic	827	95.6	23	2.7	15	1.7	865
General	12522	94.0	474	3.6	326	2.4	13322
Gynaecology	8844	96.5	230	2.5	95	1.0	9169
Neurosurgery	598	89.7	35	5.2	34	5.1	667
Ophthalmology	3768	97.7	82	2.1	8	0.2	3858
Oral/maxillofacial	2285	97.5	44	1.9	15	0.6	2344
Orthopaedic	8555	89.6	565	5.9	424	4.5	9544
Otorhinolaryngology	4803	98.1	73	1.5	19	0.4	4895
Paediatric	531	95.5	13	2.3	12	2.2	556
Plastic	1822	91.3	93	4.7	80	4.0	1995
Urology	4362	98.4	41	0.9	29	0.7	4432
Not known	18		0		0		18
Total	**48935**	**94.7**	**1673**	**3.2**	**1057**	**2.0**	**51665**

* of the total cases for the specialty; ❖ including public holidays

Table 7
Number of theatre cases (by region)

	Monday to Friday❖	%*	Saturday	%*	Sunday	%*	Total
Anglia & Oxford	4023	95.7	104	2.5	77	1.8	4204
North Thames	5784	94.1	216	3.5	147	2.4	6147
North West	7390	94.4	277	3.6	158	2.0	7825
Northern & Yorkshire	5341	94.8	173	3.1	118	2.1	5632
South Thames	5772	95.2	170	2.8	123	2.0	6065
South & West	5426	93.9	237	4.1	116	2.0	5779
Trent	4940	96.2	106	2.1	90	1.7	5136
West Midlands	5325	94.4	215	3.8	102	1.8	5642
Northern Ireland	1903	94.8	59	2.9	45	2.3	2007
Wales	3031	93.9	116	3.6	81	2.5	3228
Total	**48935**	**94.7**	**1673**	**3.2**	**1057**	**2.0**	**51665**

* of total cases from the region; ❖ including public holidays

Most (94.7%) operations were carried out between Monday and Friday.

Table 8
Theatre cases - routine and emergency (by specialty of the consultant surgeon in charge)

	Routine	Emergency	*Emergencies as %* *of total cases*
Cardiothoracic	752	113	*13.1*
General	10600	2717	*20.4*
Gynaecology	7697	1466	*16.0*
Neurosurgery	461	205	*30.8*
Ophthalmology	3712	146	*3.8*
Oral/maxillofacial	2165	176	*7.5*
Orthopaedic	6680	2861	*30.0*
Otorhinolaryngology	4744	146	*3.0*
Paediatric	440	115	*20.7*
Plastic	1529	466	*23.4*
Urology	4320	109	*2.5*
Not known	15	3	
Total	**43115**	**8523**	*16.5*

Table 8 demonstrates the specialties with the greatest number of emergency cases within this sample (general surgery, gynaecology and orthopaedic surgery). However, it is neurosurgery and orthopaedic surgery which have the highest percentages of emergency work (30.8% and 30% respectively). The presentation of this workload is unpredictable and may modify the likelihood of out-of-hours teaching and supervision by consultants in these specialities. See also figure 3 on page 61.

Tables 8 and 9 <u>exclude</u> 27 cases for which the classification of the procedure was not given.

Table 9
Theatre cases - routine and emergency (by region)

	Routine	Emergency	*Emergencies as %* *of total cases*
Anglia & Oxford	3506	693	*16.5*
North Thames	5085	1061	*17.3*
North West	6517	1307	*16.7*
Northern & Yorkshire	4636	996	*17.7*
South Thames	5078	987	*16.3*
South & West	4822	956	*16.5*
Trent	4373	754	*14.7*
West Midlands	4696	936	*16.6*
Northern Ireland	1678	329	*16.4*
Wales	2724	504	*15.6*
Total	**43115**	**8523**	*16.5*

It should be noted that the NHS Data Dictionary definitions of routine and emergency (see appendix D) are different from the clinical definitions customarily used by NCEPOD.

From Monday to Friday, there was a scheduled operating session for emergency procedures in 186 hospitals. In 182 (182/355, 51.3%) of these hospitals, the session was available between 08.00 and 18.00 hours, Monday to Friday.

Summary of time of start of emergency procedures

These data include procedures performed on public holidays.

Table 10
Specialty of consultant surgeon (emergency procedures), weekdays and weekends

	Daytime 08.00-18.00	%*	Evening 18.01-24.00	%*	Night-time 00.01-07.59	%*	Total
Cardiothoracic	68	60.2	30	26.5	15	13.3	113
General	1427	52.5	1028	37.9	260	9.6	2715
Gynaecology	742	50.6	615	42.0	108	7.4	1465
Neurosurgery	100	49.0	83	40.7	21	10.3	204
Ophthalmology	115	78.8	29	19.9	2	1.4	146
Oral/maxillofacial	107	60.8	65	36.9	4	2.3	176
Orthopaedic	1930	67.6	846	29.6	80	2.8	2856
Otorhinolaryngology	97	66.4	37	25.3	12	8.2	146
Paediatric	61	53.5	47	41.2	6	5.3	114
Plastic	283	60.7	165	35.4	18	3.9	466
Urology	60	55.1	41	37.6	8	7.3	109
Not known	3		-		-		3
Total	**4993**	**58.7**	**2986**	**35.1**	**534**	**6.3**	**8513**

* percentage of emergency procedures in the specialty

Tables 10 to 19 exclude ten cases for which the starting time of the anaesthesia or procedure was not given; hence the total number of cases analysed here is 8513, whereas the total number of emergency cases was 8523.

Table 11
Grade of the most senior surgeon present (emergency procedures), weekdays and weekends

	Daytime 08.00-18.00	%*	Evening 18.01-24.00	%*	Night-time 00.01-07.59	%*	Total
Senior house officer	671	46.5	654	45.3	119	8.2	1444
Registrar	1649	52.9	1240	39.8	229	7.3	3118
Staff grade	211	62.2	110	32.5	18	5.3	339
Senior registrar	662	58.5	390	34.5	80	7.0	1132
Clinical assistant	75	73.5	25	24.5	2	2.0	102
Associate specialist	151	65.7	67	29.1	12	5.2	230
Consultant	1425	74.6	424	22.2	61	3.2	1910
Other	28	63.6	13	29.6	3	6.8	44
Not known	121	62.4	63	32.5	10	5.1	194
Total	**4993**		**2986**		**534**		**8513**

* percentage of the total emergency procedures by the grade of surgeon

Would there be an even higher involvement of consultants if they were freed from other commitments while on emergency duty?

Table 12

Involvement of junior surgical staff in emergency procedures

	Daytime 08.00-18.00	%*	Evening 18.01-24.00	%*	Night-time 00.01-07.59	%*
Senior house officer	671	*13.4*	654	*21.9*	119	*22.3*
Registrar	1649	*33.0*	1240	*41.5*	229	*42.9*
Total	**2320**	*46.5*	**1894**	*63.4*	**348**	*65.2*

* percentage of total emergency procedures (see table 11)

These data are shown graphically in figure 7 (pages 61 to 64).

Table 13

Grade of the most senior anaesthetist present (emergency procedures), weekdays and weekends

	Daytime 08.00-18.00	%*	Evening 18.01-24.00	%*	Night-time 00.01-07.59	%*	Total
Senior house officer	1642	*49.0*	1480	*44.1*	232	*6.9*	3354
Registrar	740	*52.3*	553	*39.1*	122	*8.6*	1415
Staff grade	238	*70.2*	86	*25.4*	15	*4.4*	339
Senior registrar	359	*53.1*	253	*37.4*	64	*9.5*	676
Clinical assistant	220	*65.5*	97	*28.9*	19	*5.6*	336
Associate specialist	106	*63.1*	53	*31.5*	9	*5.4*	168
Consultant	1215	*79.3*	269	*17.6*	47	*3.1*	1531
Other	21	*58.3*	13	*36.1*	2	*5.6*	36
Not known	104	*56.2*	67	*36.2*	14	*7.6*	185
Total	**4645**	*57.8*	**2871**	*35.7*	**524**	*6.5*	**8040**
No anaesthetist present	348		115		10		473

* percentage of the total emergency cases by the grade of anaesthetist

Table 14

Involvement of junior anaesthetic staff in emergency procedures

	Daytime 08.00-18.00	%*	Evening 18.01-24.00	%*	Night-time 00.01-07.59	%*
Senior house officer	1642	*35.3*	1480	*51.5*	232	*44.3*
Registrar	740	*15.9*	553	*19.3*	122	*23.3*
Total	**2382**	*51.3*	**2033**	*70.8*	**354**	*67.6*

* percentage of total emergency procedures for which an anaesthetist was present (see table 13)

The data in table 14 are shown graphically in figure 8 (pages 61 to 64).

Tables 10 to 16 exclude ten cases for which the starting time of the anaesthesia or procedure was not given; hence the total number of cases analysed here is 8513, whereas the total number of emergency cases was 8523.

Table 15
Region (emergency procedures), weekdays and weekends
Figures in parentheses show the number of individual hospitals involved (i.e. not all hospitals reported emergency procedures).

	Daytime 08.00-18.00	%*	Evening 18.01-24.00	%*	Night-time 00.01-07.59	%*	Total
Anglia and Oxford (19)	394	56.9	261	37.7	38	5.4	693
North Thames (39)	592	55.8	383	36.1	86	8.1	1061
North West (44)	750	57.4	461	35.3	96	7.3	1307
Northern and Yorkshire (36)	623	62.6	336	33.7	37	3.7	996
South Thames (36)	573	58.1	360	36.5	54	5.5	987
South & West (28)	571	59.7	322	33.7	63	6.6	956
Trent (20)	431	57.9	262	35.2	51	6.9	744
West Midlands (36)	551	58.9	325	34.7	60	6.4	936
Northern Ireland (19)	212	64.4	97	29.5	20	6.1	329
Wales (20)	296	58.7	179	35.5	29	5.8	504
Total	**4993**		**2986**		**534**		**8513**

* percentage of the emergency procedures in the region

Table 16 (Monday to Friday)
Was the emergency procedure performed <u>during</u> or <u>outside</u> a scheduled session?

	Daytime Monday to Friday		Evening Monday to Friday	
	During	Outside	During	Outside
Cardiothoracic	35	13	2	24
General	486	529	51	753
Gynaecology	290	294	41	514
Neurosurgery	32	25	9	57
Ophthalmology	57	34	4	21
Oral/maxillofacial	46	34	5	46
Orthopaedic	911	399	74	525
Otorhinolaryngology	45	32	3	25
Paediatric	19	22	1	40
Plastic	103	72	11	107
Urology	27	23	1	32
Not known	-	3		
Total	**2051**	**1480**	**202**	**2144**

The information was not provided for 12 of the daytime cases and two of the evening cases.

Table 17 (Saturday and Sunday)
Was the emergency procedure performed <u>during</u> or <u>outside</u> a scheduled session?

	Daytime Saturday and Sunday		Evening Saturday and Sunday	
	During	Outside	During	Outside
Cardiothoracic	1	19	0	4
General	33	373	13	211
Gynaecology	14	144	3	57
Neurosurgery	1	42	0	15
Ophthalmology	3	21	0	4
Oral/maxillofacial	2	25	0	14
Orthopaedic	81	523	17	229
Otorhinolaryngology	0	19	1	8
Paediatric	0	19	1	4
Plastic	10	98	4	43
Urology	0	9	0	8
Total	**145**	**1292**	**39**	**597**

The information was not provided for 13 of the daytime cases and two of the evening cases.

Table 18 (emergency procedures <u>during</u> scheduled sessions, Monday to Friday, see table 16)
What was the type of operating theatre session?

Scheduled primarily for theatre cases planned in advance (PIA)
Scheduled primarily for emergency theatre cases (PFE)
(see appendix D for definitions)

	Daytime Monday to Friday		Evening Monday to Friday	
	PIA	PFE	PIA	PFE
Cardiothoracic	25	10	0	2
General	211	274	9	42
Gynaecology	122	168	17	24
Neurosurgery	24	8	3	6
Ophthalmology	41	16	2	2
Oral/maxillofacial	32	14	2	3
Orthopaedic	206	704	20	54
Otorhinolaryngology	26	19	0	3
Paediatric	5	14	0	1
Plastic	34	69	0	11
Urology	14	13	1	0
Total	**740**	**1309**	**54**	**148**

The information was not provided for two of the daytime cases.

Table 19 (emergency procedures <u>during</u> scheduled sessions, Saturday and Sunday, see table 17)
What was the type of operating theatre session?

  A) **Scheduled primarily for theatre cases planned in advance (PIA)**
  B) **Scheduled primarily for emergency theatre cases (PFE)**

	Daytime Saturday and Sunday		Evening Saturday and Sunday	
	PIA	PFE	PIA	PFE
Cardiothoracic	0	1	0	0
General	4	29	2	11
Gynaecology	3	11	0	3
Neurosurgery	0	1	0	0
Ophthalmology	1	2	0	0
Oral/maxillofacial	0	2	0	0
Orthopaedic	6	75	4	13
Otorhinolaryngology	0	0	0	1
Paediatric	0	0	0	1
Plastic	0	10	0	4
Urology	0	0	0	0
Total	**14**	**131**	**6**	**33**

Routine procedures

Summary of time of start of routine procedures

These data exclude 63 cases for which the starting time was not given and 10 cases for which the operation was not classified as either routine or emergency. The data include procedures performed on public holidays.

Table 20
Routine procedures by specialty of the consultant surgeon in charge (weekdays and weekends)

	Daytime 08.00-18.00	%*	Evening 18.01-24.00	Night-time 00.01-07.59
Cardiothoracic	729	96.9	10	13
General	10519	99.3	60	11
Gynaecology	7652	99.6	27	1
Neurosurgery	458	99.3	2	1
Ophthalmology	3694	99.6	13	0
Oral/maxillofacial	2155	99.6	8	1
Orthopaedic	6623	99.2	36	14
Otorhinolaryngology	4717	99.7	14	1
Paediatric	437	100.0	0	0
Plastic	1512	98.9	16	1
Urology	4292	99.5	19	1
Not known	15		0	0
Total	**42803**	**99.4**	**205**	**44**

* percentage of routine procedures in the specialty

Table 21 (Monday to Friday)
Was the routine procedure performed during or outside a scheduled session?

	Daytime Monday to Friday		Evening Monday to Friday	
	During	Outside	During	Outside
Cardiothoracic	709	10	1	9
General	10361	65	50	9
Gynaecology	7534	40	25	1
Neurosurgery	449	8	1	1
Ophthalmology	3621	12	13	0
Oral/maxillofacial	2128	11	6	1
Orthopaedic	6495	24	29	7
Otorhinolaryngology	4647	14	14	0
Paediatric	432	5	0	0
Plastic	1488	12	12	3
Urology	4225	15	19	0
Not known	15	0	0	0
Total	**42104**	**216**	**170**	**31**

Table 22 (Saturday and Sunday)
Was the routine procedure performed during or outside a scheduled session?

	Daytime Saturday and Sunday		Evening Saturday and Sunday	
	During	Outside	During	Outside
Cardiothoracic	8	2	0	0
General	76	17	0	1
Gynaecology	52	26	0	1
Neurosurgery	0	1	0	0
Ophthalmology	53	8	0	0
Oral/maxillofacial	15	1	0	1
Orthopaedic	76	28	0	0
Otorhinolaryngology	47	9	0	0
Paediatric	0	0	0	0
Plastic	8	4	0	1
Urology	37	15	0	0
Total	**372**	**111**	**0**	**4**

Table 23 (routine procedures <u>during</u> sheduled sessions, Monday to Friday, see table 21)
What was the type of operating theatre session?

Scheduled primarily for theatre cases planned in advance (PIA)
Scheduled primarily for emergency theatre cases (PFE)
(see appendix D for definitions)

	Daytime Monday to Friday		Evening Monday to Friday	
	PIA	PFE	PIA	PFE
Cardiothoracic	706	0	1	0
General	10315	18	50	0
Gynaecology	7509	10	25	0
Neurosurgery	447	1	1	0
Ophthalmology	3609	0	13	0
Oral/maxillofacial	2118	2	6	0
Orthopaedic	6375	105	28	1
Otorhinolaryngology	4630	7	14	0
Paediatric	432	0	0	0
Plastic	1477	1	11	1
Urology	4210	1	19	0
Not known	15	0	0	0
Total	**41843**	**145**	**168**	**2**

The information was not provided for 116 of the daytime cases.

Table 24 (routine procedures <u>during</u> scheduled sessions, Saturday and Sunday, see table 22)
What was the type of operating theatre session?

Scheduled primarily for theatre cases planned in advance (PIA)
Scheduled primarily for emergency theatre cases (PFE)
(see appendix D for definitions)

	Daytime Saturday and Sunday	
	PIA	PFE
Cardiothoracic	8	0
General	76	0
Gynaecology	52	0
Ophthalmology	53	0
Oral/maxillofacial	15	0
Orthopaedic	75	1
Otorhinolaryngology	47	0
Plastic	8	0
Urology	33	4
Total	**367**	**5**

Day cases (Monday to Friday 08.00 to 18.00 hrs)

These data include the procedures performed on public holidays.

19299 (45.6%) of the 42320 weekday, daytime cases classed as routine operations were described as day cases, in the specialties listed below (specialty of consultant surgeon).

368 of the 3543 cases classed as emergency procedures were described as day cases, in the specialties listed below.

Table 25
Day cases, by specialty of consultant surgeon in charge

	Routine	Emergency
Cardiothoracic	51	2
General	4572	61
Gynaecology	4305	130
Neurosurgery	20	0
Ophthalmology	1887	10
Oral/maxillofacial	1359	10
Orthopaedic	2588	97
Otorhinolarynology	1560	24
Paediatric	236	5
Plastic	735	23
Urology	1981	6
Not answered	5	0
Total	**19299**	**368**

Table 26
Day cases, by grade of the most senior surgeon present

	Routine	%	Emergency	%
Senior house officer	1682	8.7	54	14.7
Registrar	3608	18.7	123	33.4
Staff grade	1075	5.6	16	4.3
Senior registrar	1524	7.9	29	7.9
Clinical assistant	521	2.7	8	2.2
Associate specialist	668	3.5	10	2.7
Consultant	9751	50.5	121	32.9
Other	157	0.8	1	0.3
Not known	313	1.6	6	1.6
Total	**19299**		**368**	

The revolution in surgical practice is demonstrated by these figures. However, it is noteworthy that only half of the day case procedures were carried out by consultants despite the recommendations of The Royal College of Surgeons of England in 1992[1].

Table 27

Day cases, by grade of the most senior anaesthetist present

	Routine	%	Emergency	%
Senior house officer	975	6.7	75	24.0
Registrar	1453	10.1	50	16.0
Staff grade	954	6.6	17	5.4
Senior registrar	737	5.1	18	5.8
Clinical assistant	934	6.5	19	6.1
Associate specialist	791	5.5	8	2.6
Consultant	7935	54.9	117	37.5
Other	86	0.6	4	1.3
Not known	575	4.0	4	1.3
Total	**14440**		**312**	
No anaesthetist present	4859		56	

In addition, 60 procedures performed during Monday to Friday 18.01 to 23.59 were classed as day cases (54 routine, 6 emergency).

Fifteen of the routine cases were for evacuation of the products of conception (ERPC) in one hospital, between 19.00 and 21.30 hrs, described by the consultant gynaecologist as "normal working hours". Three gastroscopies were performed by a clinical assistant between 18.00 and 19.00 hrs in a hospital which had an "evening waiting list initiative gastroscopy list for people who work during the day". Four procedures for removal of wisdom teeth were carried out between 18.20 and 19.30 hrs as part of a waiting list initiative. The latest starting time for the other procedures was 20.15 hrs (extracapsular extraction of lens). The operating session had started at 13.45; the final case was the eighth on the list, finishing at 21.15 hrs. All procedures were performed by a consultant surgeon and anaesthetised, when necessary, by an associate specialist.

Three of the "emergency" day cases were ERPCs in two hospitals, between 18.45 and 19.30 hrs.

Reference

1. The Royal College of Surgeons of England. Commission on the Provision of Surgical Services. Guidelines for Day Case Surgery. Revised edition. London, March 1992.

Regional profiles

Within each region, there was a variety of types of hospitals, including those offering limited surgical specialties, and small hospitals offering only an elective, Monday to Friday service. Each hospital was classified by NCEPOD according to the median number of all types of procedures (including day surgery) reported for a weekday. In addition, the data from specialty hospitals were coded to allow separate analysis.

Tables 28 to 30 illustrate the heterogeneity of NHS hospitals. Is it good public policy, and use of resources, for surgery and general anaesthesia still to be performed in so many small hospitals?

Table 28
Classification of hospitals (NHS), including specialist hospitals

Median number of cases per weekday
up to 20
21 to 40
more than 40

Table 29
Types of hospital

Region	1-20	21-40	40+	Unable to classify*	Total
Anglia & Oxford	7	3	12	1	23
North Thames	21	16	10	1	48
North West	15	20	15	3	53
Northern & Yorkshire	11	20	8	0	39
South Thames	17	14	13	2	46
South & West	14	6	13	5	38
Trent	4	5	13	1	23
West Midlands	10	14	13	4	41
Northern Ireland	12	5	2	1	20
Wales	11	6	6	1	24
Total	122	109	105	19	355

Table 30
Number of cases (by type of hospital)

Region	1-20	21-40	40*	Unable to classify*	Total
Anglia & Oxford	360	545	3277	22	4204
North Thames	1274	2508	2362	3	6147
North West	711	2844	4162	108	7825
Northern & Yorkshire	578	2984	2070	0	5632
South Thames	772	2041	3241	11	6065
South & West	554	928	4144	153	5779
Trent	143	594	4354	45	5136
West Midlands	552	1846	3110	134	5642
Northern Ireland	733	696	574	4	2007
Wales	669	927	1626	6	3228
Total	6346	15913	28920	486	51665

* Unable to classify because only date was provided, or other data problems

Table 31
Specialist hospitals only

Specialty of hospital	Number of hospitals	Routine	Emergency	Total cases	
Cardiothoracic	5	194	34	228	
Gynaecology	6	391	57	448	
Neurosurgery	4	87	32	119	
Oncology	2	17	0	17	
Ophthalmology	9	741	53	794	
Oral/maxillofacial	2	17	1	18	
Orthopaedic	7	438	19	457	
Otorhinolaryngology	1	51	0	51	
Paediatric	8	664	164	828	
Total	**44**	**2600**	**360**	**2960**	*(5.7%)*

Table 32
Specialist hospitals, by region

		Total cases
Anglia & Oxford	2	145
North Thames	11	793
North West	9	793
Northern & Yorkshire	2	45
South Thames	4	211
South & West	3	191
Trent	3	204
West Midlands	8	509
Northern Ireland	2	69
Wales	0	0
Total	**44**	**2960**

NHS hospitals

Monday to Friday

Daytime

(08.00 to 18.00 hrs)

Monday to Friday 08.00 to 18.00 hrs (daytime)

Tables 33 to 39 cover the weekday, daytime work i.e. Monday to Friday 08.00 to 18.00 hrs. These data include procedures performed on public holidays.

There were a total of 45827 theatre cases at these times. Although the starting time was not indicated on 73 of the questionnaires, these cases were allocated to this period according to the finishing time of the procedures.

Table 33
Daytime cases (weekday), by region

	Routine cases	% of total routine cases*	Emergency cases	% of total emergency cases*
Anglia & Oxford	3471	99.0	266	38.4
North Thames	4982	98.0	401	37.8
North West	6417	98.5	511	39.1
Northern & Yorkshire	4568	98.5	441	44.3
South Thames	5010	98.7	401	40.6
South & West	4688	97.2	390	40.8
Trent	4343	99.3	319	42.3
West Midlands	4547	96.8	392	41.9
Northern Ireland	1644	98.0	153	46.5
Wales	2690	98.8	172	34.1
Total	**42360**	**98.2**	**3446**	**40.4**

* see table 9 for the denominator (total routine/emergency cases for each region). This table excludes 21 cases where the classification of the operation was not given.

Table 33 demonstrates that 98% of all routine procedures and 40% of all emergency procedures were done during the day, Monday to Friday.

Table 34 (weekday, daytime)
Specialty of consultant surgeon in charge

	Routine cases	% of total routine cases	Emergency cases	% of total emergency cases	Total	% of total cases
Cardiothoracic	719	1.7	48	1.4	767	1.7
General	10428	24.6	995	28.9	11423	24.9
Gynaecology	7590	17.9	570	16.5	8160	17.8
Neurosurgery	457	1.1	58	1.7	515	1.1
Ophthalmology	3638	8.6	89	2.6	3727	8.1
Oral/maxillofacial	2135	5.0	76	2.2	2211	4.8
Orthopaedic and trauma	6517	15.4	1268	36.8	7785	17.0
Otorhinolaryngology	4673	11.0	76	2.2	4749	10.4
Paediatric	440	1.0	43	1.2	483	1.0
Plastic	1500	3.5	170	4.9	1670	3.6
Urology	4248	10.0	50	1.4	4298	9.4
Not known	15		3		18	
Total	**42360**		**3446**		**45806**	

Table 35 (weekday, daytime)
Emergency cases as percentage of total weekday daytime cases (by specialty of consultant surgeon). Derived from table 34.

Cardiothoracic	6.3
General	8.7
Gynaecological	7.0
Neurosurgery	11.3
Ophthalmic	2.4
Oral/maxillofacial	3.4
Orthopaedic and trauma	16.4
Otorhinolaryngology	1.6
Paediatric	8.9
Plastic	10.2
Urology	1.2

Table 36 (weekday, daytime)
Grade of the most senior surgeon present

	Routine cases	% of routine cases	Emergency cases	% of emergency cases	Total	%
Senior house officer	2755	6.5	466	13.5	3221	7.0
Registrar	7274	17.2	995	28.9	8269	18.0
Staff grade	1901	4.5	174	5.1	2075	4.5
Senior registrar	3762	8.9	435	12.6	4197	9.2
Clinical assistant	766	1.8	60	1.7	826	1.8
Associate specialist	1347	3.2	114	3.3	1461	3.2
Consultant	23649	55.8	1107	32.1	24756	54.0
Other	257	0.6	23	0.7	280	0.6
Not known	649	1.5	72	2.1	721	
Total	**42360**		**3446**		**45806**	

In over 63% (28953/45806) of all operations, the consultant or senior registrar was known to be in theatre. At the time of this study, i.e. before the changes in surgical training took place, the post of surgical registrar would be held by a doctor who had spent approximately two years as a senior house officer (SHO) and who held a surgical fellowship diploma from one of the royal colleges. It is of interest that in the emergency cases, a consultant or senior registrar was present in only 44.7% (1542/3446) of the cases.

Table 37 (weekday, daytime)
Specialty of the surgical team when the most senior surgeon was a senior house officer

	Routine cases	Emergency cases	Total
Cardiothoracic	1	-	1
General	809	166	975
Gynaecology	374	137	511
Neurosurgery	8	1	9
Ophthalmic	142	5	147
Oral/maxillofacial	203	7	210
Orthopaedic and trauma	167	99	266
Otorhinolaryngology	413	6	419
Paediatric	20	2	22
Plastic	290	38	328
Urology	328	3	331
Not answered	-	2	2
Total	**2755**	**466**	**3221**

Table 38 (weekday, daytime)
Grade of the most senior surgeon present (general, orthopaedic surgery and gynaecology)

	General	%	Orthopaedic	%	Gynaecology	%
Senior house officer	975	8.5	266	3.4	511	6.3
Registrar	2158	18.9	1535	19.7	1740	21.3
Staff grade	426	3.7	415	5.3	446	5.5
Senior registrar	916	8.0	647	8.3	739	9.1
Clinical assistant	116	1.0	116	1.5	225	2.8
Associate specialist	279	2.4	394	5.1	170	2.1
Consultant	6366	55.7	4219	54.2	4156	50.9
Other	35		23		33	
Not known	156		172		144	
Total	**11427**		**7787**		**8164**	

A consultant or senior registrar was present in 62% (17043/27378) of all cases in the three largest groups of procedures. However, it is of concern that unsupervised SHOs were responsible for 13.5% (466/3446) of all emergency operations (table 36), although NCEPOD does not know their experience.

Table 39 (weekday, daytime)
Grade of the most senior anaesthetist present

	Routine cases	%*	Emergency cases	%*	Total	%*
Senior house officer	2612	7.1	936	29.3	3548	8.9
Registrar	3753	10.3	496	15.6	4249	10.7
Staff grade	2092	5.7	202	6.3	2294	5.8
Senior registrar	2073	5.7	223	7.0	2296	5.8
Clinical assistant	1930	5.3	164	5.1	2094	5.3
Associate specialist	1632	4.5	76	2.4	1708	4.3
Consultant	21272	58.1	1014	31.8	22286	56.0
General/hospital practitioner	82	0.2	9	0.3	91	0.2
Other	116	0.3	12	0.4	128	0.3
Not answered	1016	2.8	57	1.8	1073	2.7
Total	**36578**		**3189**		**39767**	
No anaesthetist present	5782		257		6039	

* percentage of cases for which an anaesthetist was present

This table shows in stark reality who, in terms of anaesthetic grades, was taking responsibility for routine and emergency cases performed in daytime working hours during 1995/96. A consultant or senior registrar anaesthetist was present in 61.8% (24582/39767) of all cases. However, for the emergency cases, only 38.8% (1237/3189) of the cases were attended by a consultant or senior registrar.

This information can be considered from a number of perspectives but, particularly when considering changes that have taken place since April 1996, the training of anaesthetists must be the most crucial. Have we grown used to a culture where "emergencies", both in anaesthesia and surgery, are too often seen as the province of the trainee?

Is the proportional decrease between routine and emergency cases managed by consultants in-hours of about one quarter sustainable for the future?

Can it be argued that SHOs taking direct responsibility for only 7.1% of routine cases but 29.3% of emergencies in-hours is justifiable in terms of the needs for their training?

Surely a fundamental reassessment of the arrangements for the management of emergency cases will be required. Emergency in-hours operating lists covered by consultant anaesthetists must be the pattern for the future, but this can only be justified if the hospital is taking sufficient acute cases to use the time of these experienced anaesthetists efficiently. From this perspective of the provision of acute cover by anaesthetists, to say nothing of the provision of surgeons, there are obvious implications for the planning of acute hospital services in the future.

NHS hospitals

Monday to Friday

Evening

(18.01 to 24.00 hrs)

Monday to Friday 18.01 to 24.00 hrs (evening)

Tables 40 to 43 cover the weekday evening work and include procedures performed on public holidays.

Table 40 (weekday evening)
Specialty of consultant surgeon

Specialty of surgeon	Routine cases	% of routine cases	Emergency cases	% of emergency cases	Total	% of total cases
Cardiothoracic	10	5.0	26	1.1	36	1.4
General	59	29.2	804	34.2	863	33.8
Gynaecology	26	12.9	555	23.6	581	22.8
Neurosurgery	3	1.5	67	2.9	70	2.7
Ophthalmic	13	6.4	25	1.1	38	1.5
Oral/maxillofacial	7	3.5	51	2.2	58	2.3
Orthopaedic and trauma	36	17.8	600	25.6	636	24.9
Otorhinolaryngology	14	6.9	28	1.2	42	1.7
Paediatric	0		41	1.7	41	1.6
Plastic	15	7.4	118	5.0	133	5.2
Urology	19	9.4	33	1.4	52	2.0
Total	**202**		**2348**		**2550**	

Of the 2550 procedures performed between 18.01 and 23.59 hrs, 522 were started between 18.01 and 19.00 hrs (i.e. start time of anaesthesia).

Table 41 (weekday evening)
Grade of most senior surgeon present

	Routine cases	%	Emergency cases	%	Total	%
Senior house officer	9	4.5	500	21.3	509	20.0
Registrar	15	7.4	969	41.3	984	38.6
Staff grade	17	8.4	99	4.2	116	4.5
Senior registrar	13	6.4	309	13.2	322	12.6
Clinical assistant	6	3.0	21	0.9	27	1.1
Associate specialist	4	2.0	48	2.0	52	2.0
Consultant	133	65.8	339	14.4	472	18.5
Other	2	1.0	11	0.5	13	0.5
Not known	3	1.5	52	2.2	55	2.2
Total	**202**		**2348**		**2550**	**100**

The procedures started between 18.01 and 19.00 hrs were performed by senior house officers (83), registrars (163), staff grades (15), senior registrars (72), clinical assistants (7), associate specialists (8), consultants (164), other (3), not answered (7).

Over 92% (2348/2550) of the cases were classed as emergencies. The routine cases would include those running over from scheduled lists which may or may not have been disrupted by emergency cases.

A consultant or senior registrar surgeon was present for only 27.6% (648/2348) of the emergency cases.

Table 42 (weekday evening)
Grade of the most senior surgeon present (general, orthopaedic surgery and gynaecology)

	General	%	Orthopaedic	%	Gynaecology	%
Senior house officer	199	23.1	59	9.3	180	31.3
Registrar	309	35.8	284	44.7	248	43.2
Staff grade	32	3.7	32	5.0	44	7.7
Senior registrar	99	11.5	108	17.0	40	7.0
Clinical assistant	6	0.7	14	2.2	4	0.7
Associate specialist	10	1.2	31	4.9	6	1.0
Consultant	192	22.2	88	13.8	40	7.0
Other	2	0.2	5	0.8	4	0.7
Not known	14	1.6	15	2.3	8	1.4
Total	**863**	**100**	**636**	**100**	**574**	**100**

The involvement of consultants and senior registrars varied in these specialties: 33.7% in general surgery, 30.8% in orthopaedic surgery and 13.9% in gynaecology.

Table 43 (weekday evening)
Grade of the most senior anaesthetist present

	Routine cases	%*	Emergency cases	%*	Total	%*
Senior house officer	16	8.8	1134	50.3	1150	47.2
Registrar	26	14.3	440	19.5	466	19.1
Staff grade	14	7.7	77	3.4	91	3.7
Senior registrar	10	5.5	192	8.5	202	8.3
Clinical assistant	1	0.6	84	3.7	85	3.5
Associate specialist	10	5.5	42	1.9	52	2.1
Consultant	94	51.6	218	9.7	312	12.8
General/hospital practitioner	0		2	0.1	2	0.1
Other	0		11	0.5	11	0.5
Not answered	11	6.0	54	2.4	65	2.7
Total	**182**		**2254**		**2436**	
No anaesthetist present	20		94		114	

* of cases for which an anaesthetist was present

Experience suggests that the way operating theatres are used during the evening makes a major contribution to the overall organisation of work. It is generally assumed that in most operating theatres operations take longer the later in the evening they take place. Delays between cases increase and in general the motivation of staff declines. This is compounded by factors such as the change over from day to night theatre shifts and that less experienced anaesthetists are managing the patients. We have no data on these matters.

Of the 43115 routine theatre cases (tables 8 and 9) considered in this report only 202 cases started after 18.00 and of these only 182 required an anaesthetist. It does not seem on this evidence that over-running of routine lists is a major problem, although there may be local exceptions. What however is clear, is that the direct involvement with cases by a consultant anaesthetist drops from 58.1% for routine cases in weekday daytime hours (table 39) to under 10% for emergencies during the evenings after 18.00, if one excludes what would appear to be over-running routine cases.

Trainees need to gain experience in handling emergency patients; once they have received basic training it is essential that they learn to take responsibility. This period in the evening is probably a very reasonable time for them to be taking on a greater proportion of the work. However, the presence of a consultant, not necessarily to give the anaesthetic, can make a major impact on the organisational aspects of the handling of cases as well as reassuring trainees that if problems arise, help is close at hand.

The specialist registrar advisors recognised the benefits of giving an anaesthetic consultant a fixed session each evening between say 17.30 and 20.30 to oversee the prompt conclusion of routine operating and the efficient organisation of emergency operating to prevent over-running late into the night.

NHS hospitals

Monday to Friday

Night

(00.01 to 07.59 hrs)

Tables 44 to 49 cover the weekday night-time work, and include procedures performed on public holidays.

Table 44 (weekday night)
Specialty of consultant surgeon

Specialty of surgeon	Routine	% of total routine cases	Emergency	% of total emergency cases	Total	%
Cardiothoracic	13	30.9	11	2.8	24	5.6
General	10	23.8	191	49.5	201	47.0
Gynaecology	1		82	21.2	83	19.4
Neurosurgery	1		12	3.1	12	2.8
Ophthalmic	0		1	0.3	1	0.2
Oral/maxillofacial	1		4	1.0	5	1.2
Orthopaedic and trauma	13	30.9	55	14.3	68	16.0
Otorhinolaryngology	1		4	1.0	5	1.2
Paediatric	0		6	1.6	6	1.4
Plastic	1		13	3.4	14	3.3
Urology	1		7	1.8	8	1.9
Total	**42**		**386**		**428**	**100**

Forty-nine of the procedures performed between 00.01 and 07.59 hrs were started between 07.00 and 07.59 hrs. Forty-one of these were routine cases which started early. 386 were emergencies and this is a small proportion of all operating.

Table 45 (weekday night)
Grade of most senior surgeon present

	00.01-06.59	%	07.00-07.59
Senior house officer	77	20.3	2
Registrar	169	44.6	3
Staff grade	14	3.7	0
Senior registrar	56	14.8	4
Clinical assistant	1	0.3	1
Associate specialist	10	2.6	0
Consultant	41	10.8	39
Other	3	0.8	0
Not known	8	2.1	0
Total	**379**	**100**	**49**

A consultant or senior registrar surgeon was present in only 25.6% (97/379) of cases which started between midnight and 06.59 hrs.

Table 46 (weekday, 00.01 to 06.59 hrs only)
Emergency procedures performed by SHO surgeons

Appendicectomy	19
Curettage of uterus/other evacuation of contents of uterus	17
Reduction/manipulation of fracture/dislocation	9
Sutures/opening of skin/operation on nail bed	9
Excision of anal polyp/drainage of ischiorectal/perianal abscess	5
Circumcision	2
Drainage of lesion of breast	2
Drainage of pilonidal sinus	2
Suture of lip	2
Autograft of skin	1
Drainage of anterior abdominal wall	1
Drainage of joint	1
Insertion of CV catheter	1
Opening of abdomen	1
Operation on ulcer of duodenum	1
Sigmoidoscopy	1
Surgical removal of tooth	1
Total	**75**

The justification for many or all of these operations at night seem dubious. It seems unlikely that consultants would have carried them out themselves had they been asked. The action of one Chief Executive who is reported to have insisted that a consultant surgeon is always present in the early hours of the morning has much to commend it.

Table 47 (weekday 00.01 to 06.59 hrs only)
Grade of the most senior surgeon present (general, orthopaedic surgery and gynaecology)

	General	%	Orthopaedic	%	Gynaecology	%
Senior house officer	41	21.8	11	20.0	17	21.8
Registrar	90	47.9	19	34.5	42	53.8
Staff grade	4	2.1	2	3.6	7	9.0
Senior registrar	22	11.7	12	21.8	7	9.0
Clinical assistant	1	0.5	0		0	
Associate specialist	2	1.1	7	12.7	0	-
Consultant	21	11.2	3		4	5.1
Other	3	1.6	0		0	
Not known	4	2.1	1		1	1.3
Total	**188**	**100**	**55**	**100**	**78**	**100**

NB the procedures performed between 07.00 and 07.59 hrs have been omitted from table 47.

The involvement of the consultant or senior registrar varied: 22.9% in general surgery, 27.3% in orthopaedic surgery and 14.1% in gynaecology.

Table 48 (weekday night)
Grade of the most senior anaesthetist present

	00.01-06.59	%*	07.00-07.59
Senior house officer	165	44.5	7
Registrar	85	22.9	7
Staff grade	12	3.2	1
Senior registrar	44	11.9	2
Clinical assistant	15	4.0	1
Associate specialist	5	1.4	2
Consultant	34	9.2	28
Other	2	0.5	-
Not answered	9	2.4	1
Total	371		49
No anaesthetist present	8		0

* percentage of cases for which an anaesthetist was present

It is accepted that operating on patients between midnight and 06.59 hrs in the absence of a clear clinical indication is neither to the benefit of the patient nor to the staff responsible for their care. The returns by surgeons, which explain the reason for timing of operations, show that about one-third of the patients were anaesthetised at this time as a result of over-stretched facilities. Either the queue for the emergency theatre built up earlier in the evening and "bumped" this case until after midnight, or the absence of an emergency theatre on the following morning resulted in a decision to operate, when on clinical grounds, the patient could have waited until daytime hours. The result was an operation taking place in a hospital where, if problems arose, support from other departments would only be at a reduced level and those in theatre carrying out the procedure were in the midst of a disturbed sleep pattern. In addition it was the time at which there was a high probability of the patient being anaesthetised by a junior trainee (SHO or registrar).

Table 49 below lists the specific procedures (total 165) managed by SHO anaesthetists between midnight and 06.59 hrs. The high number of appendicectomies, ERPCs and relatively minor orthopaedic procedures might suggest that the majority of these procedures were well within the abilities of such junior trainees. However, there were smaller numbers of more complex operations or in patients with severe co-morbidities where one might question the experience of an SHO anaesthetist as being sufficient.

The specialist registrar advisors, some themselves now consultants, were unanimous in the view that any operation carried out at this time of day by an anaesthetic trainee should only take place following discussion with a consultant. If this may not always appear essential for clinical reasons, it is only the direct involvement of consultants that will lead to the organisational changes that are needed to ensure the appropriate use of resources.

Table 49 (weekday 00.01 to 06.59 hrs only)
Emergency cases anaesthetised by SHO anaesthetists

Appendicectomy	40
Curettage of uterus/other evacuation of contents of uterus	29
Primary closed reduction of traumatic dislocation of joint/other operations or joint	10
Opening of skin/debridement of skin	9
Primary repair of inguinal hernia/femoral hernia/umbilical hernia	9
Drainage through perineal region/operation on pilonidal sinus	7
Primary open reduction of fracture of bone and intramedullary/extramedullary fixation	7
Excision of testis/operation on testis	5
Closed reduction of fracture of bone	4
Diagnostic endoscopic examination of peritoneum	4
Excision of adnexa of uterus	4
Operation on flap of skin to head or neck/autograft of skin/suture of skin	4
Total excision of colon/excision of sigmoid colon/Hartmann's operation	4
Partial excision of fallopian tube/incision of fallopian tube	3
Amputation of leg/toe	2
Drainage of lesion of breast	2
Opening of abdomen	2
Operation on Bartholin gland	2
Operation on ulcer of duodenum	2
Anastomosis of stomach to jejunum	1
Creation of ileostomy	1
Debridement of open fracture of bone	1
Drainage of anterior abdominal wall	1
Excision of lesion of anus	1
Excision of lesion of skin	1
Oesophagoscopy	1
Open drainage of peritoneum	1
Operation on epididymis	1
Operation on femoral artery	1
Operation on prepuce	1
Primary simple repair of tendon	1
Repair of subclavian artery	1
Repair of vagina	1
Surgical removal of tooth	1
Total excision of kidney	1
Total	**165**

If the justification for the list in table 46 were dubious, these seem more so. If the clinical criteria developed by NCEPOD (see below) are applied, how many of these were emergency or urgent?

Classification of operations, as defined by NCEPOD

Emergency
Immediate life-saving operation, resuscitation simultaneous with surgical treatment (e.g. trauma, ruptured aortic aneurysm). Operation usually within one hour.

Urgent
Operation as soon as possible after resuscitation (e.g. irreducible hernia, intussusception, oesophageal atresia, intestinal obstruction, major fractures). Operation usually within 24 hours.

Scheduled
An early operation, but not immediately life-saving (e.g. malignancy). Operation usually within 3 weeks.

Elective
Operation at a time to suit both patient and surgeon (e.g. cholecystectomy, joint replacment).

NHS hospitals

Saturday
and
Sunday

Saturday and Sunday

Table 50
Grade of the most senior surgeon present

	Saturday				Sunday			
	Day	Eve	Night	Total	Day	Eve	Night	Total
Senior house officer	109	80	24	**213**	93	75	16	**184**
Registrar	380	158	33	**571**	291	114	24	**429**
Staff grade	51	5	3	**59**	28	6	1	**35**
Senior registrar	164	50	13	**227**	98	33	11	**142**
Clinical assistant	37	4	0	**41**	4	0	0	**4**
Associate specialist	27	9	1	**37**	19	10	1	**30**
Consultant	422	50	11	**483**	151	36	9	**196**
Other	6	0	0	**6**	2	2	0	**4**
Not known	25	9	2	**36**	30	2	1	**33**
Total	**1221**	**365**	**87**	**1673**	**716**	**278**	**63**	**1057**

Day 08.00 to 18.00 hrs;　　　**Evening** 18.01 to 24.00 hrs;　　　**Night** 00.01 to 07.59 hrs

Table 51
Grade of the most senior anaesthetist present

	Saturday				Sunday			
	Day	Eve	Night	Total	Day	Eve	Night	Total
Senior house officer	369	188	39	**596**	308	160	25	**493**
Registrar	160	68	24	**252**	109	46	12	**167**
Staff grade	56	4	0	**60**	20	5	3	**28**
Senior registrar	72	34	5	**111**	67	27	15	**109**
Clinical assistant	50	4	2	**56**	22	9	1	**32**
Associate specialist	18	10	2	**30**	13	1	1	**15**
Consultant	367	31	10	**408**	109	20	4	**133**
Not answered	42	12	3	**57**	22	2	2	**26**
Total	**1134**	**351**	**85**	**1570**	**716**	**270**	**63**	**1003**
No anaesthetist present	87	14	2	103	46	8	0	54

Day 08.00 to 18.00 hrs;　　　**Evening** 18.01 to 24.00 hrs;　　　**Night** 00.01 to 07.59 hrs

Tables 50 and 51 confirm the findings of other studies that SHOs and registrars carry the burden of weekend work.[1]

Table 52 (Saturday)
Classification of the operation

	Day		Evening		Night		Total	%
	Rou	Em	Rou	Em	Rou	Em		
Cardiothoracic	8	12	0	1	0	2	23	1.4
General	84	214	1	128	1	46	474	28.3
Gynaecology	74	100	1	40	0	15	230	13.7
Neurosurgery	1	21	0	10	0	3	35	2.1
Ophthalmology	61	17	0	3	0	1	82	4.9
Oral/maxillofacial	15	19	1	9	0	0	44	2.6
Orthopaedic	73	347	0	133	1	11	565	33.8
Otorhinolaryngology	56	10	0	4	0	3	73	4.4
Paediatric	0	10	0	3	0	0	13	0.8
Plastic	9	51	1	28	0	4	93	5.5
Urology	36	3	0	2	0	0	41	2.5
Total	**417**	**804**	**4**	**361**	**2**	**85**	**1673**	

Day 08.00 to 18.00 hrs;   **Evening** 18.01 to 24.00 hrs;   **Night** 00.01 to 07.59 hrs

Rou = Routine; Em = Emergency (see NHS Data Dictionary definitions, appendix D).

There are planned lists on Saturdays in some hospitals.

Table 53 (Sunday)
Classification of the operation

	Day		Evening		Night		Total	%
	Rou	Em	Rou	Em	Rou	Em		
Cardiothoracic	2	8	0	3	0	2	15	1.4
General	9	198	0	96	0	23	326	30.8
Gynaecology	4	60	0	20	0	11	95	9.0
Neurosurgery	0	22	0	6	0	6	34	3.2
Ophthalmology	0	7	0	1	0	0	8	0.8
Oral/maxillofacial	1	8	0	6	0	0	15	1.4
Orthopaedic	31	266	0	113	0	14	424	40.1
Otorhinolaryngology	0	9	0	5	0	5	19	1.8
Paediatric	0	9	0	3	0	0	12	1.1
Plastic	3	57	0	19	0	1	80	7.6
Urology	16	6	0	6	0	1	29	2.8
Total	**66**	**650**	**0**	**278**	**0**	**63**	**1057**	

Day 08.00 to 18.00 hrs;   **Evening** 18.01 to 24.00 hrs;   **Night** 00.01 to 07.59 hrs

Rou = Routine; Em = Emergency (see NHS Data Dictionary definitions, appendix D).

Eighty-two percent (2241/2730) of the weekend cases were emergency procedures.

Table 54 (Saturday)
Emergency procedures - grade of most senior surgeon

	Day	%	Evening	%	Night	%	Total	%
Senior house officer	101	12.6	79	21.9	24	28.2	204	16.3
Registrar	346	43.0	157	43.5	33	38.8	535	42.8
Staff grade	19	2.4	5	1.4	3	3.5	27	2.2
Senior registrar	115	14.3	49	13.6	13	15.3	177	14.2
Clinical assistant	11	1.4	4	1.1	0		15	1.2
Associate specialist	18	2.2	9	2.5	1	1.2	28	2.2
Consultant	169	21.0	49	13.6	9	10.6	227	18.2
Other	3	0.4	0		0		3	0.2
Not answered	22	2.7	9	2.5	2	2.4	33	2.6
Total	**804**		**361**		**85**		**1250**	

Day 00.01 to 07.59 hrs   **Evening** 08.00 to 18.00 hrs   **Night** 18.01 to 24.00 hrs.

Table 55 (Sunday)
Emergency procedures - grade of most senior surgeon

	Day	%	Evening	%	Night	%	Total	%
Senior house officer	90	13.9	75	27.0	16	25.3	181	18.3
Registrar	280	43.3	114	41.0	24	38.1	418	42.2
Staff grade	17	2.6	6	2.2	1	1.6	24	2.4
Senior registrar	94	14.5	33	11.9	11	17.5	138	13.9
Clinical assistant	3	0.5	0		0		3	0.3
Associate specialist	19	2.9	10	3.6	1	1.6	30	3.0
Consultant	115	17.7	36	12.9	9	14.3	160	16.2
Other	2	0.3	2	0.7	0		4	0.4
Not answered	30	4.6	2	0.7	1	1.6	33	3.3
Total	**650**		**278**		**63**		**991**	

Day 00.01 to 07.59 hrs   **Evening** 08.00 to 18.00 hrs   **Night** 18.01 to 24.00 hrs.

Table 56 (Saturday)
Emergency procedures - grade of most senior anaesthetist

	Day	%*	Evening	%*	Night	%*	Total	%*
Senior house officer	359	47.2	186	53.4	39	47.0	584	49.0
Registrar	121	15.9	67	19.3	24	29.0	212	17.8
Staff grade	16	2.1	4	1.1	0		20	1.7
Senior registrar	69	9.1	34	9.8	5	6.0	108	9.1
Clinical assistant	29	3.8	4	1.1	2	2.4	35	2.9
Associate specialist	16	2.1	10	2.9	2	2.4	28	2.3
Consultant	118	15.5	31	8.9	8	9.6	157	13.2
Not answered	33	4.3	12	3.5	3	3.6	48	4.0
Total	**761**		**348**		**83**		**1192**	
No anaesthetist present	43		13		2		58	

Day 00.01 to 07.59 hrs   **Evening** 08.00 to 18.00 hrs   **Night** 18.01 to 24.00 hrs.

* of cases for which an anaesthetist was present

Table 57 (Sunday)
Emergency procedures – grade of most senior anaesthetist

	Day	%*	Evening	%*	Night	%*	Total	%*
Senior house officer	295	48.5	160	59.3	25	39.7	479	50.9
Registrar	108	17.7	46	17.0	12	19.0	166	17.6
Staff grade	19	3.1	5	1.9	3	4.8	27	2.9
Senior registrar	63	10.3	27	10.0	15	23.8	105	11.2
Clinical assistant	22	3.6	9	3.3	1	1.6	32	3.5
Associate specialist	12	2.0	1	0.4	1	1.6	14	1.5
Consultant	70	11.5	20	7.4	4	6.3	94	10.0
Not answered	20	3.3	2	0.7	2	3.2	21	2.2
Total	**609**		**270**		**63**		**942**	
No anaesthetist present	41		8		0		49	

Day 00.01 to 07.59 hrs   **Evening** 08.00 to 18.00 hrs   **Night** 18.01 to 24.00 hrs.

* of cases for which an anaesthetist was present

Reference

1. Wilson JA. Unsupervised surgical training: questionnaire study. Br Med J. 1997; 314: 1803-4.

igures

Figure 1

Monday to Friday - all procedures

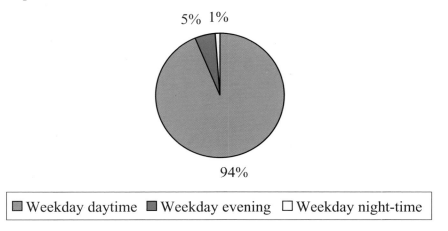

The number of procedures are given in tables 33, 40 and 44 (pages 40, 46 and 50).

Figure 2

All procedures (all days)

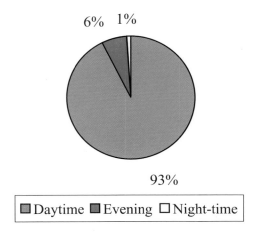

The number of procedures are given in tables 33, 40, 44 and 50 (pages 40, 46, 50 and 56).

Figure 3

Emergency procedures (all days)

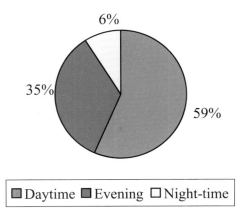

(see table 10, page 26)

Figure 4
Routine cases (all times and all days) by specialty of the consultant surgeon in charge

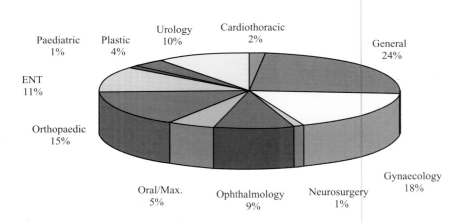

(see table 8, page 25).

Figure 5
Emergency procedures (all times and all days) by specialty of consultant surgeon in charge

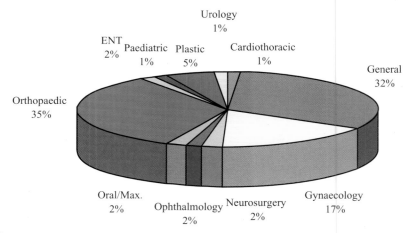

(see table 8, page 25)

Figure 6
Emergency and routine procedures, by specialty of the consultant surgeon in charge (selected specialties)

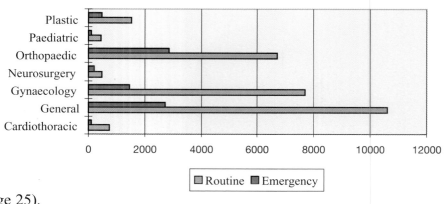

(see table 8, page 25).

Figure 7
Emergency procedures by grade of the most senior surgeon present

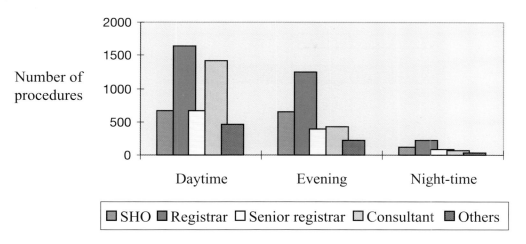

"It is the responsibility of all consultant surgeons to be involved in the management and operative care of all patients admitted under their names" (section 3.6 "Emergency Surgery" in The Senate of Surgery of Great Britain and Ireland, Consultant Surgical Practice and Training in the UK, June 1997).

Figure 8
Emergency procedures by grade of the most senior anaesthetist present

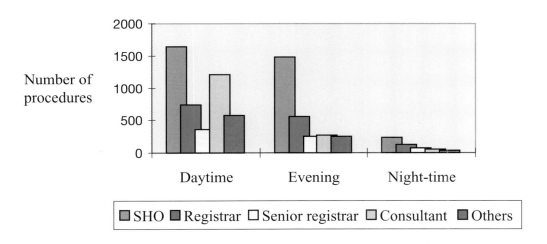

(see table 14, page 27)

The Royal College of Anaesthetists recognises that by the end of the SHO stage, to be ready for a specialist registrar post, anaesthetists should be able to "organise, with the surgical team, an emergency list; identify potential problems and seek appropriate help" (The Royal College of Anaesthetists. Specialist Training for Senior House Officers in Anaesthesia). To obtain this experience requires guidance from those more senior. The high proportion of cases managed by SHOs on their own both during the day, in the evening and at night would appear to suggest that the needs of service are overwhelming the needs of training.

Figure 9
Emergency procedures during/outside scheduled sessions

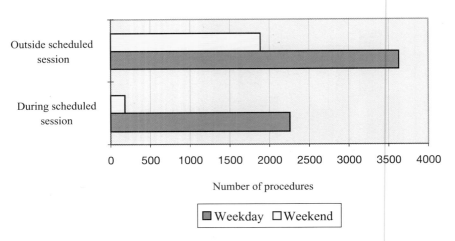

(See tables 16 and 17, pages 28 and 29)
The definitions of scheduled sessions and type of operating theatre session are given in Appendix D

Figure 10
Emergency procedures performed during scheduled sessions (see figure 9) /type of operating theatre session

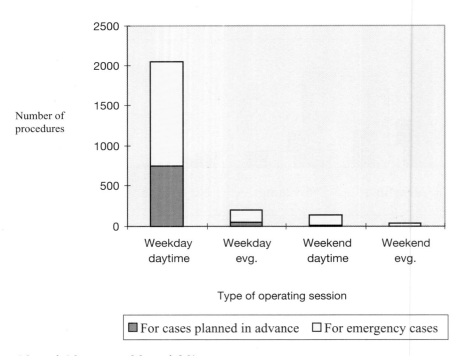

(See tables 18 and 19, pages 29 and 30).

Why operate then?

Requests were sent to consultant surgeons for further information about 5408 of the procedures performed out-of-hours (as defined by NCEPOD, see page 13). Replies were received about 4031 (74%) cases (reminder letters were not sent). All replies were coded according to the reasons for the timing of the procedure.

ROUTINE PROCEDURES

Monday to Friday (evening and night)

Nineteen of the 174 replies mentioned clinical reasons for the timing of the procedure. Other reasons (which may be multiple for each case) were:

Normal working hours	66
Evening list for private patients	23
Over-running list	23
Waiting list initiative	14
GP fundholders' list	5
Queuing for theatre space	5
Trauma list	2
No reason stated (i.e. form returned blank)	7

Replies from two hospitals mentioned twilight operating lists (e.g. 18.30 to 21.30 hrs) to maximise the use of theatre time. The elective operating list in a new spinal unit started regularly at 07.00 hrs, until 17.00 hrs. At another hospital, there were three operating sessions per day, between 07.30 and 19.00 hrs.

The following specific comments were included in the responses:

"I do not have access to theatre except between 17.30 and 21.00 on a Friday evening"
(Three cases from a spinal injuries consultant working in a specialist orthopaedic hospital)

"The operation began at 18.20 as the elective list had been interrupted by an emergency case at 16.00 until 17.50 (a leaking aneurysm). This occurs as there is no emergency theatre in this hospital."
(Hysterectomy and salpingo-oophorectomy, patient aged 35)

"As there was an intensive care bed I elected to operate on this patient after hours rather than cancel him."
(CABG in a specialist cardiothoracic hospital, 19.00 to 20.50 hrs)

"We have to frequently work late to keep up with the clinical workload and tend to put additional cases on the consultant's list."
(Endoscopy followed by sigmoidoscopy at 18.06 and 18.23 hrs by consultant)

Saturdays (any time)

Ten of the 293 replies mentioned clinical reasons for the timing of the procedure. Other reasons (which may be multiple for each case) were:

Waiting list initiative	150
Normal working hours	56
Private patients	35
GP fundholders' list	21
No other time available/queuing for theatre space	7
Weekend trauma list	3
No reason stated (i.e. form returned blank)	3

One hospital was a day surgery unit, operating six days per week for elective surgical cases. Another hospital had a routine Saturday morning list. The replies about six procedures on a GP fundholder's list commented that the theatre was "specially provided by the hospital" to treat patients who had been on the waiting list for more than one year. In another hospital, a "staff grade list" for gynaecology was arranged for a Saturday morning when a consultant was available in the hospital.

The following specific comments were included in the responses:

"The patient had been scheduled on a routine list on the previous day but was displaced by more urgent/deserving cases so was put on a list on Saturday morning."
(Debridement and skin graft of tibial wound by consultant plastic surgeon)

"Patient admitted from fracture clinic on previous day, for reduction. Space not available until after midnight, so postponed until following morning."
(MUA little finger and percutaneous reduction of fracture by consultant orthopaedic surgeon)

Sundays (any time)

Ten of the 24 replies mentioned clinical reasons for the timing of the procedure. Other reasons (which may be multiple for each case) were:

Private patients	4
Waiting list initiative	3
No other time available	2
Normal hours	1
Weekend trauma list	1

The following specific comments were included in the responses:

"Admitted with epigastric pain. OGD revealed oesophagitis? It suited the theatre staff to do this procedure on a Sunday."
(Oesophagoduodenoscopy by a general surgical registrar, followed by another OGD for weight loss)

"Acute GI bleed admitted at weekend and Monday was a bank holiday. Therefore performed as a "planned emergency" as further delay until next list was not clinically satisfactory."
(Gastroscopy performed by a surgical registrar at 13.00 hrs; patient admitted on 28-12-95, procedure on 31-12-95)

"The plastic surgery department does not have access to a morning emergency operating list."
(Primary simple repair of tendon and application of plaster cast by senior registrar in plastic surgery, at 14.20 hrs)

EMERGENCY PROCEDURES

Monday to Friday (any time)

1305 of the 2001 replies mentioned clinical reasons for the timing of the procedure. Other reasons (which may be multiple for each case) were:

Queuing for theatre space	354
No emergency theatre available during the day	155
No list space available	43
Normal trauma list	27
No reason stated in the patients' notes	19
Surgeon committed elsewhere earlier in the day	15
Transferred from another hospital	13
Normal working hours	11
Over-running list	11
Convenience	8
Anaesthetist not available earlier	4
Delay in getting patient to theatre	2
Error in decision-making	2
Private patient	1
Request from physician	1
No reason stated (i.e. form returned blank)	77

The following specific comments were included in the responses:

"The on-take team had an outpatients clinic all afternoon. When it finished around 5.30 pm the emergency case still had to take its turn with all the emergencies in orthopaedics, gynaecology, urology etc."
(Appendicectomy at 21.35 hrs by general surgical registrar)

"Patient was brought to theatre at 08.00 for emergency list but nurses had fed patient at 07.30, therefore had to be cancelled until later that day"
(Debridement of right foot by general surgical registrar at 22.00 hrs)

"Failure of management to acknowledge need for daytime emergency theatre and personnel to be available."
(ERPC by registrar at 22.00 hrs)

"Patient attended A&E department 3-8-95 at 11.20 pm and was not fasted. Trauma list on 4-8-95 am was fully booked already. No trauma list on 4-8-95 pm and more urgent cases operated on between 6.00 pm and 9.30 pm."
(Repair of radial nerve by orthopaedic consultant at 21.40 hrs)

"As a more general point we are struggling badly to provide emergency theatres in daytime hours. I have a personal audit of the problem."
(Subcutaneous fasciotomy, monitoring of pressures by general surgical registrar at 21.10 hrs)

"Only one patient can be operated on at a time after 5.00 pm due to limited theatre staff, only one anaesthetist is on call. Emergency theatre not available 9.00 am to 5.00 pm."
(Incision and drainage of axillary abscess by general surgical registrar at 01.45 hrs)

"Patient admitted as emergency. Performed, as per traditional way, at the end of the day by a junior doctor and this is frequently inappropriate. I am personally campaigning to change this outmoded system. I believe that the operation should have been done in normal hours in an emergency theatre by a consultant."
(Repair of inguinal hernia with mesh prosthesis by general surgical registrar at 23.35 hrs)

"The child got to theatre 7 hours after the injury and this is a less than average delay, but by no means an ideal situation."
(Primary suture and graft for oblique amputation of thumb tip by SHO plastic surgeon at 20.23 hrs, patient aged 4 years)

"Routine to carry out suitable cases until 11.00 pm. Operations generally carried out by consultants as junior staff now no longer capable of such procedures due to decreased training because of hours reduction"
(Appendicectomy at 21.15 hrs)

"We have asked for a dedicated evening emergency list but funding is not available."
(Exploration of wound on wrist by SHO plastic surgeon at 18.51 hrs)

"Duty registrar did not follow departmental recommendations about start time for non-urgent trauma admissions."
(Right ambi hip screw at 00.05 hrs)

"Medically should have waited until the following morning but would then have had to compete with other emergencies."
(Laparotomy, division of adhesions and revision of ileostomy by consultant general surgeon at 20.55 hrs; patient admitted nine days previously)

"Because the organisation for transplantation is chaotic and shambolic. With more careful planning there is no reason whatsoever why the operation could not have been performed in daylight hours."
(Heart transplant by consultant cardiac surgeon at 21.30 hrs)

"The only trauma lists available are Monday morning and Friday afternoon. There is too much demand on these sessions."
(Two cases - exploration of wound and repair of leg muscle and bimalleolar fracture of right ankle by orthopaedic registrar at 20.55 and 19.01 hrs on a Thursday)

"Patient waited for nearly 30 hours for this procedure. Lack of operating theatre time - theatres busy with general surgical cases. Accumulation of plastic surgery emergency cases."
(Exploration and suture of hand wound by SHO plastic surgeon at 01.08 hrs)

"Admitted 01.30 hrs; hospital not on take but ambulance diverted in from journey to A&E in another hospital in group when patient lost blood pressure. Team called in from home and case started at 02.40 hrs."
(Repair of ruptured aortic aneurysm by consultant general surgeon).

"Patient admitted at 03.00 hrs and the viability of the bowel in the hernia was in doubt; urgent surgery indicated. An elective theatre list was available starting at 08.30 hrs but this was very full. No emergency theatre for general surgery during that day."
(Primary repair of femoral hernia at 05.00 hrs by a general surgical registrar)

"We would like to have an early pregnancy diagnosis and treatment unit (with operating theatre) but it has been said that our numbers do not warrant it."
(ERPC by registrar at 20.20 hrs)

"There is no trauma list and no twilight operating session and rarely will a second theatre be opened."
(Washout of left shoulder by orthopaedic registrar at 23.30; patient admitted on previous day)

"Why operate then?"

Saturdays (any time)

576 of the 805 replies mentioned clinical reasons for the timing of the procedure. Other reasons (which may be multiple for each case) were:

Queuing for theatre space	67
Normal trauma list	47
No emergency theatre available during the day	23
No list space available	14
Normal working hours	8
Convenience	8
Transferred from another hospital	7
Private patient	4
Surgeon committed elsewhere earlier in the day	2
Request from physician	1
No reason stated (i.e. form returned blank)	50

The following specific comments were included in the responses:

"Fractured necks of femur are frequently operated on at weekends."
(Right DHS by staff grade surgeon from 12.00 to 14.45 hrs)

"Elective admissions cancelled through lack of beds. Elective list utilised for emergency procedure."
(Fem-pop bypass and debridement of foot by consultant general surgeon at 09.35 hrs)

"Referred from emergency medical service 11-7-95. Treated conservatively, planned for trauma list 14.7.95 but insufficient space on list. Cancelled second time."
(Incision of olecranon bursa by orthopaedic registrar at 14.05 hrs on 15.7.95)

"Over 60% of all trauma cases at this hospital are operated on outside the normal working day. There are no trauma lists as such; each of 8 consultants have one session a week to cope with the trauma requirements of a local population of 900,000."
(Open reduction and internal fixation of lateral malleoli by orthopaedic registrar at 10.00 hrs)

"Theatre space available during the day for emergencies but often unavailable 4.30 to 6.30 pm because of reduction in nursing staff from 5.00 to 5.30 pm, reduction in the number of ODAs and tea break 6.00 to 6.30 pm."
(Cleaning and suturing of wound by orthopaedic registrar at 19.08 hrs)

"From October we will do all non-urgent trauma during the daytime lists. This has occurred because of pressure from the consultants to have such a list."
(DHS for fractured neck of femur by orthopaedic registrar from 17.35 to 19.55 hrs)

Sundays (any time)

562 of the 735 replies mentioned clinical reasons for the timing of the procedure. Other reasons (which may be multiple for each case) were:

Normal trauma lists	59
Queuing for emergency theatre	59
No emergency theatre during daytime	18
No list space available	5
Normal working hours	3
Transfer from another hospital	3
Over-running lists	2
Convenience	1
No reason given (i.e. form returned blank)	40

The following specific comments were included in the responses:

"It is exceptional for theatre facilities to be available for such cases during normal working hours. I would that it were otherwise"
(Appendicectomy by SHO in general surgery, with SHO anaesthetist, at 18.56 hrs)

"Our hospital has a trauma list 9.00 am to 5.00 pm, 365 days per year and 5.30 to 9.00 pm Tuesday and Thursday, and still patients have to wait sometimes."
(Primary open reduction of fracture of long bone, grade of surgeon not provided, at 10.20 hrs)

"We have 4 trauma lists per week, but they are used for elective cases that have been on the waiting list for nearly a year. There is pressure from management to shorten waiting lists."
(DHS by registrar at 14.49 hrs)

"This was a weekend; if it had been a weekday he would have had to wait until the evening as there are no weekday daytime trauma sessions."
(Debridement of left middle finger tip amputation by senior registrar in plastic surgery at 10.00 hrs)

"Why operate then?"

Personal
Commentaries

Personal commentary - Dr G S Ingram MBBS FRCA

Critical mass

Successful outcome for patients after surgery is dependent on teamwork between medical and other professional staff together with management. It is also dependent on the structures within which the team works. Together this grouping needs to be of such size and ability as to ensure a sufficient depth of experience to undertake the care of the more severely ill patients, even when things are not going well. A hospital needs to have a certain "critical mass" of activity. Technically brilliant surgery may increase the chances of a favourable outcome but, with major operations, that alone will not guarantee success. Traditionally the surgeon, having direct responsibility for the patient, has been dominant in deciding most aspects of the organisation and timing of the surgical operation. Today these decisions are increasingly being affected by limitations on resources, as well as the organisation within which the team works. This may, for instance, be the lack of an ICU or HDU bed, or insufficient theatre staff to open an additional emergency theatre. These result in cancellation or delay of the patient's operation.

Resources, ultimately financial, are likely to be an ever-increasing limitation on clinical practice. It is therefore necessary that when considering the information gathered in this report, and looking to the future, fundamental questions be asked about current arrangements. This will enable appropriate planning to make the best use of those resources that are available.

NCEPOD in previous reports about patients who die has sought to discourage the practice of night-time operations with inexperienced staff. But it is recognised that there will always patients who need, on the basis of clear clinical indications, to have their operations at such times. The question is how many patients fall into this category where clinical indications alone, not disorganisation in the system, are the reason for operations taking place in the middle of the night.

Operations on Monday to Friday at night, in the information collected, represented 0.83% of the total operations (428 of 51,665 in NHS hospitals). However, included in this 428 were 40 routine cases started between 07.00 and 07.59; deducting these, the true percentage of cases is 0.75%. This represents cases currently being carried out but to what extent are these all absolutely necessary? Some of the indications seem questionable. The written replies from surgeons indicated that many operations took place within these hours either because there was no theatre available earlier (as a result of the build-up of urgent cases) or because, if the patient were not operated on, there would be unacceptable further delay (because there was no provision for an emergency theatre the following morning). The provision of staffed emergency theatres available throughout the full 24 hours must be the goal for all major hospitals. The number of emergency and urgent cases will inevitably fluctuate, but on the evidence available in this report an attempt can be made to examine on what basis such provision can be justified.

It appears therefore that the proportion of operations that need to be performed at night in an emergency theatre from Monday to Friday will be about one half of one percent of the total workload. To take as an arbitrary starting point the premiss that at least one operation should be performed each weekday night if such a fully staffed theatre is to be justified then almost 200 operations would need to be performed each weekday. In table 29, page 36, only 105 of the 355 hospitals even exceeded 40 per weekday. It has to be acknowledged that there are other factors, for instance the presence of separate specialist units and in some parts of the country geographical distances, which may make it necessary to modify this premiss. But there are also other cogent reasons why the concentration of activity makes good sense.

If the operations that take place at night are occasioned by clinical indications alone, and because of the size of the hospital they are taking place in significant number, then other facilities will need to match this demand. An appropriately staffed recovery room can be available, the provision for HDU beds might be such that patients operated on at these times can be managed there postoperatively, or in the case of the more severely ill they can be stabilised in an ICU preoperatively as well as returned there postoperatively. The care of paediatric patients undergoing surgery requires experienced nursing and medical staff. Twenty-three of the patients operated on between midnight and 07.59 were children under the age of five. Concentration of emergencies facilitates arrangements for their surgery and anaesthesia.

That 65% of operating surgeons and 67% of anaesthetists managing patients at night were junior trainees (SHOs or Registrars), may be of concern not just on grounds of experience. The hours that junior doctors can work continues to be reduced even since the information was collected for this report. It is unlikely that they will be able to contribute to the out-of-hours provision to the same degree in the future. If consultants are to take a greater involvement then this commitment will have to recognised within their sessional provision and used effectively. This surely means concentration in emergency and urgent cover.

To achieve such "critical mass" may mean that as well as emergency and urgent patients presenting at, and being referred to such larger hospitals, other patients who develop complications that require further surgery will need to be transferred to these larger hospitals from smaller units. The current provisions for the transfer of patients in all circumstances is unsatisfactory, as has been indicated in previous NCEPOD reports. Improvements are possible to make such transfers safe and will be essential if these concepts are to be developed.

In order to provide a comprehensive, rational and efficient emergency service hospitals will have to work together. It has been suggested that a population base of 450-500,000 is the ideal model for the organisation of healthcare[1]. Hospitals serving smaller populations will have to link their services if appropriate specialist expertise is to be available together with the increasingly expensive technological equipment that is required for the investigation and care of surgical patients. It is no longer possible to base an emergency service solely on the presence of junior trainees in surgery and anaesthesia working unacceptably long hours.

Reference

1. The Senate of Surgery of Great Britain and Ireland. Consultant Surgical Practice and Training in the UK. London, June 1997.

Personal commentary - Mr C D Collins MA ChM FRCS

The training implications for surgeons of out-of-hours operating

The 1995/96 NCEPOD study reports on the timing of surgery and this overview concentrates on the training implications of out-of-hours surgery. Previous reports[1,2] suggested that many such operations were carried out by unsupervised anaesthetists and surgeons in training with sub-optimal results.

This study of 51,665 operations demonstrated that in fact only 6.1% of cases were operated on out-of-hours of which a significant number were carried out on planned extra trauma or waiting list initiative operating lists either in the evenings or at weekends. Whilst such elective utilisation of operating time is to be commended for service provision, it raises concerns for training as it is clear from this study that these lists are not training opportunities for junior surgeons as they are usually carried out by staff surgeons and at times when trainee surgeons are off-duty.

Apart from early starts and late finishes of routine daytime elective lists, most of the remaining out-of-hours surgery is carried out on emergencies.

Emergencies present one of the most challenging and demanding aspects of surgical practice[3] and yet, as the Audit Commission[4] points out, whilst elective surgery is organised and led by consultants, emergency surgery is led by the trainee who decides if and when to request more senior and experienced assistance. This clearly creates the risk that inappropriate responsibility will be taken by junior surgical trainees who may not be able to obtain more senior assistance for either the assessment of or the operation on an emergency because the consultant is committed to other programmed activity such as an operating list or an out-patient clinic. Furthermore the trainee might feel obliged not to trouble their more senior colleague at the weekend or particularly during the night time hours of midnight to 7.00am. That this latter risk was not realised is shown by detailed analysis of the 77 emergency procedures undertaken by an SHO without more senior supervision between 00.01 and 07.59 hrs (weekdays) which showed that appendicectomy and evacuation of contents of uterus comprised 36 of the 77 cases with only two other procedures regarded as probably requiring more senior assistance.

This study breaks down the out-of-hours emergency surgery not only into weekday night time (00.01 to 07.59 hrs) but also evenings (18.01 to 24.00 hrs) and Saturdays and Sundays. The most senior surgeon present in the operating theatre in each of these three latter periods was: consultant in 14.4%, 18.2% and 16.2% respectively and SHO in 21.3%, 16.3% and 18.3% with registrar, senior registrar staff surgeons for the remainder.

Furthermore, during week daytime (08.01 to 18.00 hrs) consultants were only involved in about one third of the emergency operations carried out. Whilst this might have been due to lack of availability, the low incidence of consultant involvement in the evenings and at weekends represent missed opportunity for hands-on teaching which, whilst possibly less necessary in 1995/96, will now, in 1997, be essential in order to actively train the more junior trainee surgeons in the new (Calman) shortened training scheme.

Both the Royal College of Surgeons of England[5] and the Senate of Surgery[3] recommend that the emergency surgical service should be led by consultants whose responsibility it is then to actively delegate clinical and operative care to their juniors to a degree appropriate to their level of confidence and competence. Consultants should be free of all other programmed duties for the duration of their emergency on call period in order to fulfil this responsibility. In order for this to be achieved cost effectively, there would need to be many more consultants working in units large enough to deploy a rota of consultants on emergency duty only with 24-hour fully staffed operating theatres available for them to use for the benefit of the patient and the surgical trainee.

Whilst such organisational changes may take considerable time to achieve in some hospital units and the increase in the number of consultants will be slow, it is important that as more consultants are appointed and therefore the frequency of on-call commitment diminishes, consultants should involve themselves more in the hands-on teaching opportunities and care of emergencies to the point where it can truly be said that the emergency service in all surgical specialties is led not by the junior surgical trainee but by the consultant whose responsibility it is.

References

1. Campling EA, Devlin HB, Lunn JN. The Report of the National Confidential Enquiry into Perioperative Deaths 1989. NCEPOD, London 1990.

2. The Report of the National Confidential Enquiry into Perioperative Deaths 1993/94. NCEPOD, London 1996.

3. The Senate of Surgery of Great Britain and Ireland. Consultant Surgical Practice and Training in the UK. London, June 1997.

4. Audit Commission. The Doctor's Tale Continued. The audits of hospital medical staffing. HMSO, 1996.

5. The Royal College of Surgeons of England. The Provision of Emergency Surgical Services - An Organisational Framework. RCS, London, June 1997.

Personal commentary - Professor L Strunin MD FRCA FRCPC

Preoperative starvation in emergent and urgent cases

The normal stomach empties a clear fluid load within minutes,[1] but solid material depending on its nature may take several hours. These observations led to a routine practice of starving elective patients from midnight on the night prior to an operation in the belief that the stomach would be empty when the patient presents for anaesthesia the following day. The risk of aspiration of stomach contents into the lungs either during induction of anaesthesia, before the airway could be protected, or during emergence from anaesthesia was thus thought to be reduced. However, withholding of fluids for prolonged periods has been shown to be unnecessary in elective patients.[2] The recent Practice Guidelines from the American Society of Anesthesiologists (1997)[3] which are based on a systematic review of the literature between 1940-1996, recommend that the minimum fasting period for clear liquids should be two hours regardless of the age of the patient. The Guidelines further note that there is no evidence that the routine use of gastrointestinal stimulants (metoclopramide), gastric secretion blockers (cimetidine, famotidine, ranitidine, omeprazole, lansoprazole), antacids (sodium citrate, sodium bicarbonate, magnesium, trisilicate), antiemetics (droperidol, ondansetron) or anticholinergics (atropine, scopolamine, glycopyrrolate) will prevent pulmonary aspiration in elective patients. The situation may be entirely different in patients with gastrointestinal disease, following trauma and/or the administration of opioids or other drugs, alcohol ingestion or pregnancy all of which may dramatically lengthen the ability of the stomach to empty. For obvious reasons there are no controlled studies to determine how long this delay might be. If such patients have consumed solid material and then require an anaesthetic for an operation the question arises how long should one wait? In the face of life or limb threatening disease it is usual to accept that the surgical imperative overrides the risk of aspiration and providing the patient is adequately resuscitated with regard to fluid and/or blood products as required the problem of the full stomach may be considered as follows:

a) A gastric secretion blocker should be given intravenously if time permits, remembering they take about 45 minutes to be effective. Oral non-particulate antacids are effective immediately but increase gastric volume and may not mix well in the full stomach. It should be noted that there are no studies to show that such pharmacological manoeuvres will, in any particular patient, either prevent pulmonary aspiration or reduce its potentially damaging effect.

b) The airway should be assessed and if there is an anticipated major difficulty then consideration should be given to a local or regional technique if appropriate. However, if these fail general anaesthesia may still be required.

c) Is an awake tracheal intubation appropriate? The disposition of the patient, skill of the anaesthetist and availability of suitable equipment will dictate whether this is the best course.

d) If general anaesthesia is the option then:

    i)   suitable large bore intravenous lines should be established under local anaesthesia.

    ii)   monitoring consistent with the degree of patient illness or injury should be established, but must include pulse oximetry and the availability of immediate end tidal carbon dioxide measurement.

    iii)   a range of cuffed endotracheal tubes, laryngoscopes, introducers, other aids to tracheal intubation and a powerful suction should be available.

    iv)   the patient should be preoxygenated.

    v)   intravenous induction with a short acting barbiturate or propofol followed by suxamethonium (rapid sequence induction using pressure[4]) will provide the best conditions for tracheal intubation. If there are contraindications to suxamethonium then a large dose of a short acting non-depolarising agent should be given. Cricoid pressure requires a dedicated assistant who understands the relevant anatomy. Compressing the oesophagus between the cricoid (from the Greek meaning a ring - the cricoid is the only complete tracheal cartilaginous ring and lies immediately below the thyroid cartilage) and the vertebral body behind will prevent regurgitation, but there is some concern that in the face of active vomiting continued pressure could result in oesophageal rupture. A further problem is that enthusiastically applied cricoid pressure may distort the larynx and make tracheal intubation impossible. Cricoid pressure should be maintained after tracheal intubation until end tidal carbon dioxide monitoring demonstrates unequivocally that the tube is in the trachea and the endotracheal cuff has been inflated. If the trachea cannot be intubated, cricoid pressure should be maintained, consideration should be given to allowing the patient to awaken, or if surgery is really imperative, can an airway be maintained with a simple oral device and the patient turned into the lateral position if appropriate?

For the patient where there is not an immediate surgical urgency anaesthetists have usually delayed for the time that they believe the normal stomach will empty solid material i.e. four to six hours (it is interesting to note that the American Society of Anesthesiologists Practice Guidelines recommend eight hours). However, there are anecdotal tales of patients producing solid material 24 hours after ingestion - the classic example being the individual who eats and drinks well, gets into an evening fracas, ends up with a fractured jaw and now presents a dilemma for the anaesthetist (a potentially difficult airway and a full stomach) even if the operation is delayed till the following morning. Often these delays move the operation outside the normal working hours and add the potential of other unquantifiable risks in relation to the availability of skilled help for the anaesthetist and the level of expertise and training of the anaesthetic and surgical team. It may well be that these emergent and urgent operations should either be done immediately (since a short time delay of a few hours cannot guarantee an empty stomach) and treated as life or limb threatening and the risk of pulmonary aspiration accepted or the cases should be delayed to the following day for a 'routine' emergency session. This type of decision requires senior surgical and anaesthetic input and available 'emergency time' in the operating theatres during the working day. Previous NCEPOD reports support the latter view.

Mendelson[5] reviewed retrospectively the records of 44,016 pregnant patients from his hospital between 1932 and 1945. He noted 66 cases of aspiration of stomach contents into the lungs. In 45 cases, he was able to determine the aspirated material; in 40 it was liquid and the patients developed the characteristic chest radiographic changes of Mendelson's syndrome (acid aspiration syndrome). However, it is important to note that none of these patients died. Five patients inhaled solid material and died, in Mendelson's opinion from suffocation. In the same paper Mendelson described some rabbit studies designed to elucidate the cause of the radiographic changes. He found that injection of normal saline or distilled water at volumes of 5ml/kg into the rabbit's trachea was harmless. However, when he took gastric aspirate from his patients and acidified it with hydrochloric acid and injected this into his rabbits he observed the same chest radiographic changes he had seen in his patients. Neutralised vomitus was not harmful, unless it contained solid material which led to either partial obstruction with ensuing massive atelectasis or complete obstruction and suffocation. As a result of his observations, Mendelson offered the following advice for management of obstetric patients:

1. No oral feeding during labour - i.v. fluids should be given.

2. Wide use of local anaesthesia for operative obstetrics.

3. Alkalinization and emptying of the stomach before general anaesthesia.

4. Competent administration of general anaesthesia with full appreciation of the dangers of aspiration during induction and recovery from anaesthesia.

Good advice even after 50 years.

Roberts and Shirley,[6] on the basis of a single experiment in an anaesthetised monkey proposed that a volume of greater than 25ml (i.e. 0.4ml/kg in a 70kg human) with a pH of less than 2.5 aspirated into the lungs was potentially harmful. More recent work in monkeys [7, 8] suggests that 0.8ml/kg and a pH approaching 3.5 is required before harm occurs. Clearly such studies cannot ethically be conducted in humans. Nevertheless it is interesting to speculate why none of Mendelson's patients died, despite probably having aspirated considerably greater amounts of fluid than in these experimental studies. By contrast, the triennial *Confidential Enquiries into Maternal Deaths in the United Kingdom* detail with depressing regularity such deaths over the past twenty years. Other factors such as repeated attempts at tracheal intubation despite obvious hypoxia and the use of positive pressure ventilation after inhalation of gastric contents may be responsible. The concept of reducing the residual gastric volume (RGV) to 25ml or less and raising the pH above 2.5 has passed into the anaesthetic literature as a desirable feature of preoperative preparation to prevent acid aspiration. Is this achievable in patients by starvation? The simple answer is no. The longer fluid is with-held in general the larger the RGV and the lower the pH. The American Society of Anesthesiologists Practice Guidelines also show that drugs are similarly not a guarantee of either reducing RGV or raising pH to 'safe' values in a particular patient. Indeed experimentally aspirated particulate antacids from the stomach into the lungs cause damage independent of volume or pH.

References

1. Hunt JN. Some properties of an alimentary osmoreceptor mechanism. Journal of Physiology (London) 1956; 132: 267-288.

2. Strunin L. How long should patients fast before surgery? Time for new guidelines. British Journal of Anaesthesia 1993; 70: 1-3.

3. Practice Guidelines for Preoperative Fasting and Use of Pharmacologic Agents for Prevention of Pulmonary Aspiration: Application to Healthy Patients Undergoing Elective Procedures. A report by the American Society of Anesthesiologists 1997.

4. Sellick BA. Cricoid pressure to control regurgitation of stomach contents during induction of anaesthesia. Lancet 1961; ii: 404-406.

5. Mendelson CL. The aspiration of stomach contents into the lungs during obstetric anesthesia. American Journal of Obstetrics and Gynaecology 1946; 52: 191-205.

6. Roberts RB, Shirley MA. Reducing the risk of acid aspiration during Cesarian section. Anesthesia and Analgesia 1974; 53: 859-868.

7. Raidoo DM, Rocke DA, Brock-Utne JG, Marszalek A, Engelbrecht HE. Critical volume for pulmonary acid aspiration: reappraisal in primate model. British Journal of Anaesthesia 1990; 65: 248-250.

8. Rocke DA, Brock-Utne JG, Rout CC. At risk of aspiration: new critical values of volume and pH? Anesthesia and Analgesia 1993; 76: 666-669.

Personal commentary - Professor D J Leaper MBChB MD ChM FRCS FRCSEd

Professor Leaper was provided with the data shown on pages 84 to 87.

Diagnosis and management of appendicitis

The diagnosis of appendicitis is essentially a clinical, preoperative decision, usually based on signs and symptoms coupled with a degree of experience (which is difficult to measure the acquisition of and be sure of being adequate). Nevertheless, a negative appendicectomy rate (no histological proof of inflammation) remains at approximately 20%, with an incidence of perforation at the same level. Clearly these figures appear to be too high as the morbidity, and rare mortality, after appendicectomy are significant and require regular audits of diagnostic accuracy and outcomes. Most complications are infectious, or are related to adhesions or wound failure.

The indications of inflammation, pulse rate, pyrexia and white cell count, are not discriminants for acute appendicitis. A low haemoglobin on routine testing may indicate an underlying, confusing and coincident disease process such as chronic inflammatory bowel disease or a distal cancer which must not be ignored. Plain X-rays are rarely helpful as the signs of appendicitis are so non-specific and there is probably no place for their routine use. The once popular but invasive use of techniques such as peritoneal microbiology and cytology have not become established. All other imaging techniques such as scintigraphy,[1] MRI,[2] CT scanning,[3] and ultrasound,[4, 5] have been used. The advantages of the latter investigation are most obvious, being non-invasive and portable with an accuracy of 80-90%, and associated with leading to low negative appendicectomy rates.

Several computer-based or simple algorithms have been devised but have not gained widespread use or have been found not to work in other surgical centres or other countries. Few scoring systems improve the diagnostic accuracy of more senior clinicians but could be useful to surgeons in training; the Alvarado score is probably the best.[6, 7] Biochemical markers of inflammatory disease such as proteases, free radicals and interleukins have been considered and C reactive protein correlates well with acute appendicitis but is usually too slow to be helpful for diagnosis.[8]

In the elderly and in young children there is a higher rate of perforation, possibly related to a poor or underdeveloped immune response. In these patients there is also a higher chance of an atypical presentation with the attendant risk of a missed diagnosis. Appendicitis can mimic almost every other abdominal (or thoracic) condition including diseases usually classified as being 'medical' rather than surgical. Barium studies may help in diagnosis or exclude other diseases, particularly those in the elderly such as a distal cancer or diverticulitis, which may be the cause of an acute appendicitis even if rare.[9] The use of midline incisions for a laparotomy to treat appendicitis (and exclude distal obstructions) has not been consistently justified, whereas histological examination of all appendices is logical. Suspicion of appendicitis at the extreme ages of life must remain high.

Delay by the patient and delay in diagnosis to surgery does seem to matter, with an attendant increase in the number of appendiceal perforations.[10, 11, 12] In general terms, however, there appears to be no risk in waiting several hours to operate on a daytime emergency list provided that the patient does not have generalised peritonitis, signs of spreading inflammation or has another complicating feature (e.g. in children or pregnancy). It is not acceptable to operate out of hours in other circumstances.[13]

Audit at the author's institution has confirmed this but this NCEPOD report shows that up to 50% of appendicectomies are undertaken between 6.00pm to midnight and up to 10% after midnight (see page 84). Any waiting time (overnight) allows full resuscitation, correction of any clinical instability, rehydration and the institution of thromboembolic and antibiotic prophylaxis. The same audit shows that two thirds of all appendicectomies are safely undertaken by SHO/registrar surgeons and anaesthetists.

Delay in children is not appropriate as perforation rates reach 39% at 24 hours and 54% at 36 hours.[14] Similarly in pregnancy delay should not follow a firm diagnosis. Appendicitis is the commonest non-obstetric need for laparotomy during pregnancy and should be undertaken early to avoid perforation and a subsequent foetal loss of 20%.[15]

In non pregnant women laparoscopy has a part to play. In an audit at the author's institution laparoscopy was unhelpful in men but did exclude gynaecological diseases in women thereby avoiding needless appendicectomy. Other studies have been even more positive and indicate that progression to laparoscopic appendicectomy is easy and safe [16, 17, 18, 19] with less wound infections and a shorter postoperative stay. Many more audits will be published in this field but need to answer two questions: whether open appendicectomy can be replaced by the laparoscopic technique (which is currently unacceptable in training programmes) and whether the incidence of adhesions, with increase of the theoretical risk of infertility, can be reduced (by a long term random controlled trial).

There have been trials of conservative treatment of acute appendicitis but there is an unacceptable rate of recurrence or complications.[20] Nevertheless, it seems that giving appropriate antibiotic prophylaxis at diagnosis is reasonable although proof from a random controlled trial is needed. If the delay to surgery is too long 'prophylaxis' may need to be prolonged. Prophylaxis to cover aerobes and anaerobes, and given parenterally (preferably IV) at induction of anaesthesia is associated with the lowest rates of postoperative infectious complications.[21] In the presence of perforation and peritonitis prolongation to three or five days of therapy should be considered.

Appendicectomy is a safe operation with a low morbidity and mortality. It has been traditionally an important training operation which can safely be undertaken by supervised SHO and registrar trainees. It would be a pity to lose this operation entirely from basic surgical training to laparoscopic higher training, particularly if the incidence of appendicitis continues to fall. Operations can almost always be deferred to daytime operating lists except in the very young and old, in pregnancy or when there is generalised or rapidly spreading peritonitis. On these occasions senior surgical and anaesthetic staff should be involved anyway. The practice of incidental appendicectomy during operations for other conditions should be avoided as it carries an unacceptable rate of infectious complications.

References

1. Evetts BK, Foley CR, Latimer RG, Rimkus DS. TC-99 hexamethyl propyleneamine oxide scanning for the detection of acute appendicitis. J Am Coll Surg 1994; 179: 197-201.

2. Incescu L, Coskun A, Selcuk MB, Akan H, Sozubir S, Bernay F. Acute appendicitis: MR Imaging and sonographic correlation. Am J Roentgenol 1997; 168: 669-674.

3. Lane MJ, Katz DS, Ross BA, Clautice-Engle TL, Mindelzun RE, Jeffrey RB. Unenhanced helical CT for suspected acute appendicitis. Am J Roentgenol 1997; 168: 405-409.

4. Zoller WG, Kellner H, Schwerk WB. Value of ultrasound in diagnosis of acute appendicitis. Bildgebung 1996; 63: 78-82.

5. Zeidan BS, Wasser T, Nicolas CG. Ultrasonography in the diagnosis of acute appendicitis. J Roy Coll Surg Ed 1997; 42:24-26.

6. Ohmann C, Yang Q, Franke C. Diagnostic scores for acute appendicitis. Eur J Surg 1995; 161: 273-281.

7. Calder JDF, Gajraj H. Recent advances in the diagnosis and treatment of acute appendicitis. Br J Hospital Med 1995; 54: 129-133.

8. Paajanen H, Mansikka A, Laato M, Kettunen J, Kostianinen S. Are serum inflammatory markers age dependent in acute appendicitis. J Am Coll Surg 1997; 184: 303-308.

9. Bizer LS. Acute appendicitis is rarely the initial presentation of cecal cancer in the elderly patient. J Surg Oncol 1993; 54: 45-46.

10. Walker SJ, West CR, Colmer MR. Acute appendicitis: does removal of a normal appendix matter, what is the value of diagnostic accuracy and is surgical delay important? Ann Roy Coll Surg Eng 1995; 77: 358-363.

11. Murphy E, Mealy K. Timing of operation for appendicitis. Br J Surg 1997; 84: 1004-1005.

12. Eldar S, Nash E, Sabo E, Matter I, Kumn J, Mogilner JG, Abrahamson J. Delay of surgery in acute appendicitis. Am J Surg 1997; 173: 194-198.

13. Campling EA, Devlin HB, Hoile RW, Lunn JN. The Report of the National Confidential Enquiry into Perioperative Deaths 1990. London 1992.

14. Chande VT, Kinnane JM. Role of the primary care provider in expediting care of children with acute appendicitis. Arch Ped Adolesc Med 1996; 150: 703-706.

15. Al-Mulhim AA. Acute appendicitis in pregnancy. Int Surg 1996; 81: 295-297.

16. Cox MR, McCall JL, Padbury RT, Wilson TG, Wattchow DA, Toouli J. Laparoscopic surgery in women with a clinical diagnosis of acute appendicitis. Med J Aus 1995; 162: 130-132.

17. Tronin RJ, Burova VA, Grinberg AA. Laparoscopic diagnosis of acute appendicitis in women. J Am Ass Gynecologic Laparoscopists 1996; 3: 257-261.

18. Hallfeldt K, Puhlmann M, Waldner H, Sweiberer L. Diagnostic problems in acute appendicitis and indications for laparoscopic appendicectomy. Lang Archiv fur Chir 1996; 113: 553-555.

19. Chiarugi M, Buccianti P, Celona G, Decanini L, Martino MC, Goletti O, Cavina E. Laparoscopic compared with open appendicectomy for acute appendicitis. Eur J Surg 1996; 162: 385-390.

20. Eriksson S, Granstrom L. Randomised controlled trial of appendicectomy versus antibiotic therapy for acute appendicitis. Br J Surg 1995; 82: 166-169.

21. Leaper DJ, Pritchett CJ. Prophylactic antibiotics in general surgical practice. Current Practice in Surgery 1989; 1: 178-184.

Personal commentary - Professor L Spitz and R Surana

Professor Spitz was provided with the data shown on pages 84 to 87.

The management of acute appendicitis in infants and children

Acute appendicitis is one of the most common surgical emergencies in paediatric practice. Despite major improvements in the overall management of the condition, it remains responsible for a small but significant mortality and a substantial morbidity. There may be a considerable delay in establishing the diagnosis, particularly in the young infant (<2 years), and overall there is a 10-20% false positive diagnostic error.

Diagnosis

The diagnosis of an acute appendicitis in children is usually relatively clear following a careful history and thorough physical examination. The classical presentation is of periumbilical pain radiating and localising in the right iliac fossa associated with tenderness and guarding, and nausea and vomiting. In patients in whom the diagnosis was inconclusive, a period of active observation is recommended. The diagnosis may be particularly difficult in the pre-school age group and in adolescent girls. Recently, ultrasonography and contrast computerised tomography have been advocated as additional diagnostic investigations while laparoscopy may be particularly useful in the adolescent female.

Preoperative management

The infant with perforated appendicitis rapidly becomes fluid and electrolyte depleted and requires vigorous resuscitation prior to surgery. The remainder, unless there has been prolonged delay in diagnosis, generally do not require special resuscitation. Perioperative antibiotics are invaluable in reducing the risk of complications.

Surgery

Timing

Prompt surgery for suspected perforated appendicitis is the accepted treatment of choice. Where there is a diagnostic doubt a period of active observation is recommended. There is no evidence that this management protocol increases the morbidity of appendicitis in children. The need to carry out surgery in the middle of the night has been questioned. The risk of developing complications when the procedure is delayed until the following morning is not increased.

Setting

The Royal College of Anaesthetists, the Association of Paediatric Anaesthetists and the British Association of Paediatric Surgeons recommend that children under the age of 3 years should be referred to specialist centres unless the local hospital has an appropriately trained general surgeon and anaesthetist provided with all the facilities required for the conduct of surgery in children.

Surgeon

As a result of recent changes in the training programme, the Basic Surgical Trainees will not be competent to carry out appendicectomies independently. In the early years of higher surgical training it will be necessary for the consultant to be present at the operation. Restricting the procedure when feasible to the working day will facilitate the presence more often of a consultant in the operating theatre.

Technique

The approach of choice is a short Lanz, muscle-splitting incision. Careful and meticulous technique will be rewarded with an improved outcome. Drains are generally unnecessary and primary wound closure is preferred.

Conclusion

Early and accurate diagnosis, adequate preoperative preparation and prompt, safe surgery remain the cornerstones of management of acute appendicitis in childhood. This will result in a reduced perforation rate, avoidance of unnecessary surgery and a reduction in the morbidity (and mortality) of acute appendicitis.

Selected references

1. Jones PF. Active observation in the management of acute abdominal pain in childhood. Br Med J 1976; ii: 551-553.

2. Surana R, Quinn F, Puri P. Is it necessary to perform appendicectomy in the middle of the night in children? Br Med J 1993; 306: 1168.

Appendicectomy (adults[*])

These data include the following procedures:

H01   Emergency excision of appendix
H02   Other excision of appendix

The total number of procedures analysed was 450.

Table 57
Time of start of anaesthesia

	Monday to Friday	Saturday and Sunday
08.00 to 18.00 hrs (daytime)	142	65
18.01 to 24.00 hrs (evening)	142	41
00.01 to 07.59 hrs (night-time)	48	12
Total	332	118

Table 58
Grade of the most senior surgeon present

Monday to Friday

	Daytime 08.00 to 18.00 hrs	Evening 18.01 to 24.00 hrs	Night-time 00.01 to 07.59 hrs
Senior house officer	46	50	14
Registrar	46	69	24
Staff grade	3	3	1
Clinical assistant	1	-	-
Senior registrar	12	9	4
Associate specialist	3	4	1
Consultant	23	6	1
Not answered	8	1	3
Total	142	142	48

Saturday and Sunday

	Daytime 08.00 to 18.00 hrs	Evening 18.01 to 24.00 hrs	Night-time 00.01 to 07.59 hrs
Senior house officer	17	16	7
Registrar	33	13	5
Staff grade	2	-	-
Clinical assistant	-	1	-
Senior registrar	7	6	-
Associate specialist	1	3	-
Consultant	2	2	-
Not answered	3	-	-
Total	65	41	12

---

[*] aged 16 years and above

Table 59

Grade of the most senior anaesthetist present

Monday to Friday

	Daytime 08.00 to 18.00 hrs	Evening 18.01 to 24.00 hrs	Night-time 00.01 to 07.59 hrs
Senior house officer	67	93	29
Registrar	18	24	7
Staff grade	8	5	1
Senior registrar	4	5	4
Clinical assistant	9	3	-
Associate specialist	-	-	2
Consultant	32	11	3
Not answered	4	1	2
Total	**142**	**142**	**48**

Saturday and Sunday

	Daytime 08.00 to 18.00 hrs	Evening 18.01 to 24.00 hrs	Night-time 00.01 to 07.59 hrs
Senior house officer	45	25	8
Registrar	6	7	2
Staff grade	2	1	-
Senior registrar	6	5	-
Clinical assistant	-	-	1
Associate specialist	1	-	-
Consultant	3	3	-
Not answered	2	-	1
Total	**65**	**41**	**12**

Appendicectomy (children[*])

These data include the following procedures:

H01   Emergency excision of appendix
H02   Other excision of appendix

The total number of procedures analysed was 239.

Table 60
Time of start of anaesthesia

	Monday to Friday	Saturday and Sunday
08.00 to 18.00 hrs (daytime)	56	43
18.01 to 24.00 hrs (evening)	93	26
00.01 to 07.59 hrs (night-time)	18	3
Total	**167**	**72**

Table 61
Grade of the most senior surgeon present

Monday to Friday

	Daytime 08.00 to 18.00 hrs	Evening 18.01 to 24.00 hrs	Night-time 00.01 to 07.59 hrs
Senior house officer	21	28	5
Registrar	18	37	12
Staff grade	-	5	-
Senior registrar	6	10	1
Associate specialist	1	1	-
Consultant	10	8	-
Not answered	-	4	-
Total	**56**	**93**	**18**

Saturday and Sunday

	Daytime 08.00 to 18.00 hrs	Evening 18.01 to 24.00 hrs	Night-time 00.01 to 07.59 hrs
Senior house officer	12	8	2
Registrar	22	13	-
Senior registrar	5	-	1
Associate specialist	2	1	-
Consultant	1	4	-
Not answered	1	-	-
Total	**43**	**26**	**3**

---

[*] aged up to and including 15 years

Table 62
Grade of the most senior anaesthetist present

Monday to Friday

	Daytime 08.00 to 18.00 hrs	Evening 18.01 to 24.00 hrs	Night-time 00.01 to 07.59 hrs
Senior house officer	18	55	10
Registrar	8	14	5
Staff grade	2	3	2
Senior registrar	5	4	
Hospital practitioner	2	-	-
Clinical assistant	3	4	1
Associate specialist	1	-	-
Consultant	17	8	-
Not answered	-	5	-
Total	56	93	18

Saturday and Sunday

	Daytime 08.00 to 18.00 hrs	Evening 18.01 to 24.00 hrs	Night-time 00.01 to 07.59 hrs
Senior house officer	21	17	3
Registrar	10	4	-
Staff grade	1	-	-
Senior registrar	5	1	-
Clinical assistant	2	-	-
Associate specialist	-	1	-
Consultant	4	3	-
Total	**43**	**26**	**3**

Fractures of the femoral neck and intertrochanteric fractures

The records relating to the four codes listed below were analysed separately, according to the grade of the most senior surgeon in theatre and also the time of the day and the day of the week.

W19.1	Pin and plate or DHS	378
W24.1	Reduction cervical fracture and pin or screw fixation	31
W47.1	Primary cementless hemiarthroplasty	47
S48.1	Primary cemented endoprosthesis	15

Table 63
Grade of the most senior surgeon present

Monday to Friday

	Daytime 08.00 to 18.00	Evening 18.01 to 24.00	Night-time 00.01 to 07.59	Total
SHO	21	1	0	22
Registrar	90	15	2	107
Staff grade	24	6	0	30
Senior registrar	40	2	1	43
Clinical assistant	6	4	0	10
Associate specialist	72	5	0	77
Consultant	1	2	0	3
Other	1	2	0	3
Not answered	14	0	0	14
Total	**269**	**37**	**3**	**309**
				(295 answers)

Saturday and Sunday

	Daytime 08.00 to 18.00	Evening 18.01 to 24.00	Night-time 00.01 to 07.59	Total
SHO	15	3	0	18
Registrar	57	8	0	65
Staff grade	8	0	0	8
Senior registrar	25	3	2	30
Clinical assistant	3	0	0	3
Associate specialist	6	1	0	7
Consultant	6	0	0	6
Not answered	3	0	0	3
Total	**123**	**15**	**2**	**140**
				(137 answers)

During weekdays there was an average of 66 cases/day, whereas at the weekends this average was 70/day. The weekends do not seem overburdened. Should these cases be done at the weekend? The answer is that they should be done as soon as the patient is fit, and not delayed for operational reasons. As they present evenly over the week, they should have their surgery distributed the same way. However, the weekend staffing levels should recognise this need in a planned manner, not the customary context of surgical extemporisation that so often obtains at weekends, due to inappropriate resource allocation.

Of all the cases, 375 (86%) were operated upon during the daytime period and only 14% in the evenings or at night. This 14% figure should be reduced. There should be dedicated operating theatre time for these vulnerable patients. Out-of-hours operating, with often unfamiliar staff, both nursing and anaesthetic, is suboptimal.

Consultants were present at only 1% of weekday procedures and only 4% at weekends! There can be no justification for this. These patients have a life-threatening injury, often associated with other risk factors and deserve care delivered by experienced senior surgeons. Who is teaching the trainees?

At the other end of the spectrum, only 9.3% were operated upon by SHOs. The remaining operations were performed by either higher surgical trainees (56%) or non-consultant career grades (30%). Many of these will be experienced in this type of procedure.

A picture emerges of a service undertaken largely during the daytime hours, with no weekend emphasis, but virtually totally unsupervised by consultants.

The ideal model is a dedicated proximal femoral fracture service, seven days a week, not competitive with the vagaries of acute skeletal trauma, either in terms of theatre allocation, nursing levels or senior surgical staff. An example of such an approach is the Peterborough hip fracture service, which has achieved outstanding outcomes. Some other centres have arranged dedicated operating time for hip fractures, but sadly they are few, as yet.

These goals, regrettably, are probably not widely achievable so long as:-

1. surgical trainee working hours are unrealistically restricted,
2. the health authorities blackmail the trusts to displace acute work in order to satisfy elective targets, irrespective of medical need and
3. consultants do not allocate sufficient priority in this clinical arena, either to their elderly patients or to their trainees.

Only when the senior orthopaedic establishment gives to these patients the importance that they deserve and takes the necessary effective and uncomfortable political action at both local and national levels shall we be justifiably proud of the service that we render them.

Personal commentary - Professor P M S O'Brien MBBCh MD FRCOG

The management of early pregnancy loss

This topic has recently been reviewed by the National Medical Advisory Committee of the Scottish Office Department of Health (1996) [ref.] and the 33rd Study Group of the Royal College of Obstetricians and Gynaecologists on the 29 April and 1 May 1997 (report to be published on 6 November 1997). Both groups agreed that the way forward was for all Departments of Obstetrics and Gynaecology to set up Early Pregnancy Assessment Units with access to readily available diagnostic and treatment facilities. They also recognised the special medical and psychological needs of women with early pregnancy loss, either miscarriage or ectopic pregnancy, and considered that these Units should be situated in a dedicated area of the Obstetric and Gynaecology accommodation. It was recommended that provision should also be made for appropriate counselling and support and the implications for subsequent fertility were highlighted.

Early pregnancy units should establish protocols and criteria for the medical and surgical management of miscarriage. On medical grounds most surgical evacuations for retained products of conception can wait for a number of hours, which is of course why they tend to be put at the end of the emergency theatre queue. It would be preferable for there to be ready access to theatre time which is more likely to occur in a Maternity Theatre. However, the emotional and psychological needs of the women concerned cannot be underestimated when cases are managed in the proximity of women with ongoing pregnancies.

The expectant management of incomplete miscarriage and medical management of miscarriage can only be considered where arrangements are in place for follow-up and prompt access to operating facilities.

Ectopic pregnancies are increasingly being dealt with by laparoscopic surgery and only where there is evidence of acute haemorrhage or shock need laparotomy be undertaken. The urgency of the operation is clearly a matter for clinical judgement but it is true that many ectopic pregnancies can be managed electively, particularly now that earlier diagnosis is common and the urgency minimised. In consideration of the laparoscopic management of ectopic pregnancy, videoo equipment should be available and provision must be made for the training of medical and nursing staff in its use. Similarly, gynaecological units should institute facilities for the clinical management and training in laparoscopic treatment of ectopic pregnancy.

Early pregnancy units should have the necessary facilities for the diagnosis of early pregnancy including access to abdominal and transvaginal ultrasound and rapid, sensitive hCG assays.

The magnitude of the problem and associated issues cannot be underestimated as at least 10-15 percent of all pregnancies result in spontaneous loss of the products of conception. Even the development and advent of (a) non-surgical methods such as mifipristone and prostaglandins for uterine evacuation (b) the use of non-intervention techniques for the diagnosis of tubal pregnancy plus (c) the use of laparoscopic surgery in the management of ectopic pregnancy will not reduce the need for theatre time. The aim must be to place the surgical management of early pregnancy problems on scheduled daytime lists, designated emergency theatre lists or during dedicated time on routine lists.

Reference

The Scottish Office Department of Health. The management of early pregnancy loss. November 1996.

Review of the deaths (anaesthetic and surgical questionnaires)

Review of the deaths (anaesthetic questionnaires)

The data presented in the following section relate to anaesthetic questionnaires returned for patients who were included in this survey and who subsequently died within 30 days of the operation. It is therefore effectively a random sample of deaths following anaesthesia.

In all, 508 deaths were identified and anaesthetic questionnaires were sent out for 450 cases. Of these, 280 were returned and the overall return rate was 62.2%. All returned questionnaires were examined by the specialist registrar advisors who commented on those which they believed included remediable factors.

These patients were for the most part elderly and in poor preoperative health. They were, in terms of the anaesthetic challenge they presented, likely to be amongst the more difficult that anaesthetists had to manage. Their deaths were usually inevitable; anaesthesia and surgery were interventions that attempted to slow rather than prevent this outcome.

Those who died were more likely in comparison with the whole sample to have an anaesthetic given by a senior registrar (11.1% against 6.1%) and marginally more likely for it to be given by a consultant (57.5% compared with 51.3%). Otherwise for training grades there was little difference.

Much of the information is identical to that in previous NCEPOD reports but in examining these cases the specialist registrar advisors drew attention to a number of issues.

- **Decision-making** was still considered to be unsatisfactory in some cases; too many decisions are made by too junior trainees. The specialist registrar advisors were strongly of the opinion that a decision to operate should be made by consultants.

- **Preoperative management** was sometimes poor. Guidance from experienced staff was needed in resuscitating patients, and on occasions this may require referral to an ICU preoperatively. A rush to operate before adequate resuscitation was completed was likely to lead to prolonged and often unproductive postoperative intensive care.

- **Management of intravenous fluids** was poor in some cases. There are benefits and dangers in their use. On occasions a lack of fundamental understanding of physiology appeared to be the problem.

- **Records and charts** were often poorly kept or inadequate.

Deaths (anaesthetic questionnaires)

Table A1
Hospital type

DGH or equivalent	187
University/teaching	79
Surgical specialty	11
Other acute/partly acute	2
Independent	1
Total	**280**

Table A2
Proxy anaesthetists

Chairman of division	7
College tutor	5
Duty consultant	44
Other consultant	20
Other	11
Total	**87**

Table A3
Special care areas in the hospital in which the operation took place (answers may be multiple)

Recovery area or room equipped and staffed for this purpose	272
High dependency unit (HDU)	114
Intensive care unit (ICU)	261
Other	13

Table A4
Restrictions on admission of patients to the recovery area after anaesthesia

None	236
Not available in all locations	6
Closed at night	35
Closed at weekends	10
Other restriction	7

Table A5
Restrictions on admission of patients to HDU after anaesthesia

None	70
Closed at night	2
Closed at weekend	6
Available only for certain categories of patient	21
No HDU available in the hospital	166
Other	16
Not answered	3

(Total number of cases where an HDU was available in the hospital = 117)

Table A6
Restrictions on admission of patients to ICU after anaesthesia

None	184
Only ventilated patients admitted	5
Available only for certain categories of patient	13
Shortage of beds/nursing staff	55
Not answered	5

Table A7
Grades of all anaesthetists who were present at the start of this anaesthetic

Senior house officer (SHO)	116
Registrar	74
Staff grade	10
Clinical assistant	7
Associate specialist	8
Consultant	161
Other	1

Table A8
Most senior anaesthetist present at the start of the operation

		%
Consultant	161	*57.5*
Registrar	34	*12.1*
Senior house officer	33	*11.8*
Senior registrar	31	*11.1*
Associate specialist	8	*2.9*
Clinical assistant	7	*2.5*
Staff grade	6	*2.1*

Table A9
Year of first full-time anaesthetic training post - SHOs anaesthetising alone

1963	1
1982	1
1984	1
1987	1
1988	2
1989	1
1990	1
1991	1
1992	2
1993	3
1994	8
1995	5
Not answered	6

Table A10
Higher diploma(s) in anaesthesia held by the most senior anaesthetist present at the start of the operation

None	11
Fellowship	198
DA (or part 1 FRCA)	62
Part 2 FRCA	34
Other	22
Not answered	10

Table A11
Was the most senior anaesthetist employed in a locum capacity?

Yes	19
No	258
Not answered	3

If yes, grade of locum

Senior house officer	1
Registrar	5
Senior registrar	2
Consultant	10
Associate specialist	1

If yes, was this locum post part of a recognised training programme (trainee grades only)?

Senior house officer	no	1
Registrars	yes	1
	no	4
Senior registrar	yes	1
	no	1

The locum SHO anaesthetist had been in post for 1 year and 2 months. The SHO and registrar posts were not accredited by the Royal College of Anaesthetists.

Deaths (anaesthetic questionnaires)

Table A12
Did the anaesthetist seek advice at any time from another anaesthetist (not mentioned in question 7)?

Yes	49
No	220
Not answered	11

Grades of most senior anaesthetist	Grade from whom advice sought	
Senior house officer	Registrar	3
Senior house officer	Registrar and consultant	3
Senior house officer	Consultant	6
Senior house officer	Staff grade	2
Registrar	Registrar	1
Registrar	Senior registrar	1
Registrar	Senior registrar and consultant	1
Registrar	Consultant	13
Senior registrar	Senior registrar	1
Senior registrar	Consultant	5
Consultant	Senior registrar	2
Consultant	Consultant	4
Staff grade	Consultant	1
Associate specialist	Consultant	2
Clinical assistant	Consultant	4

Table A13
Did any colleague (not mentioned earlier) come to help at any time?

Yes	32
No	227
Not answered	21

Grades of most senior anaesthetist	Grade who came to help	
Senior house officer	Senior house officer	1
Senior house officer	Registrar and consultant	1
Senior house officer	Consultant	3
Senior house officer	Staff grade	1
Registrar	Senior house officer	1
Registrar	Senior house officer and consultant	1
Registrar	Registrar	1
Registrar	Consultant	3
Senior registrar	Senior house officer	1
Senior registrar	Registrar	1
Senior registrar	Senior registrar	1
Senior registrar	Consultant	2
Consultant	Senior house officer	2
Consultant	Registrar	4
Consultant	Senior registrar	3
Consultant	Consultant	6

Table A14
Age of patient

0 to 10	2
11 to 20	2
21 to 30	3
31 to 40	1
41 to 50	12
51 to 60	19
61 to 70	62
71 to 80	92
81 to 90	72
91+	15
Total cases	**280**

Table A15
Was the patient transferred from another hospital?

Yes	36
No	242
Not answered	2

If yes, had the patient's condition apparently deteriorated during transfer?

Yes	3
No	23
Not answered	10

Table A16
Classification of the operation

Emergency	44
Urgent	124
Scheduled	75
Elective	32
Not answered	5

Table A17
Was a record of the patient's height and weight available?

Weight

Yes	116
No	162
Not answered	2

Height

Yes	32
No	243
Not answered	5

Table A18
Was an anaesthetist consulted by the surgeon (as distinct from informed) before the operation?

Yes	147
No	121
Not answered	12

Table A19
Did the anaesthetist visit the patient before the operation?

Yes	265
No	8
Not answered	7

If yes, where?

Ward	212
Outpatient department	2
Accident & Emergency department	8
ICU/HDU	38
Other	9

Was this anaesthetist present at the start of the operation?

Yes	245
No	12
Not answered	8

Table A20
Investigations done before the anaesthetic

None	3
Haemoglobin	273
Packed cell volume (haematocrit)	212
White cell count	256
Sickle cell test	6
Blood group +/- cross match	215
Coagulation screen	113
Plasma electrolytes - Na	258
- K	247
- Cl	84
- HCO_3	106
Blood urea	253
Creatinine	242
Serum albumin	153
Bilirubin (total)	135
Glucose	164
Amylase	45
Urinalysis	106
Blood gas analysis	66
Chest X-ray	203
Electrocardiography	244
Respiratory function tests	16
Special cardiac investigation	32
Special neurological investigation	32
Others relevant to anaesthesia	32

Table A21
Coexisting medical diagnoses

None	20
Respiratory	100
Cardiac	160
Neurological	56
Endocrine	50
Alimentary	57
Renal	51
Hepatic	22
Musculoskeletal	27
Vascular	43
Haematological	37
Obesity	12
Sepsis	36
Other	39
Not answered	4

Table A22
ASA status

1	3
2	48
3	104
4	101
5	19
Not answered	5

Table A23
Measures taken to reduce gastric acidity and volume, as prophylaxis against acid aspiration

None	165
Antacids	9
H_2 antagonists	43
Metoclopramide	26
Proton pump inhibitor	9
Nasogastric/stomach tube	48
Other	19
Not answered	4

Table A24
Did the patient receive intravenous fluid therapy in the 12 hours before induction?

Yes	174
No	102
Not answered	4

Table A25
Were measures taken to improve or protect the cardiorespiratory system before induction of anaesthesia?

Yes	152
No	119
Not answered	9

If yes, measures taken:

Antibiotic therapy	76
Bronchodilators	32
Diuretics	46
Inotropes or vasoactive drugs	40
Cardiac resuscitation	3
Chest physiotherapy	39
Airway management	32
Steroids	10
Pleural aspiration	1
Oxygen therapy	70
Other	32

Table A26
Were premedicant drugs prescribed?

Yes	78
No	200
Not answered	2

If yes, drugs prescribed:

Atropine	3
Diazepam	5
Fentanyl	3
Hyoscine	6
Lorazepam	7
Metoclopramide	24
Midazolam	3
Morphine	8
Papaveretum	3
Pethidine	4
Temazepam	37
Promethazine	2
Non-steroidal analgesics	1
Other	21

Table A27
Was non-invasive monitoring established just before the induction of anaesthesia?

Yes	268
No	5
Not answered	7

If yes, monitors:

Electrocardiogram	239
Blood pressure	221
Pulse oximetry	262
Capnography	55
Inspired oxygen	72
Temperature	16
Other	8

Table A28
Was <u>invasive</u> monitoring established <u>before</u> inductionof anaesthesia?

Yes	84
No	188
Not answered	8

If yes, monitors:

Central venous pressure	64
Arterial line	70
Pulmonary arterial line	16
Blood gas analysis	38
Other	3

Table A29
Were any measures taken (before, during or after operation) to prevent venous thrombosis?

Yes	181
No	90
Not answered	9

If yes, which?

	Before or during	After
Aspirin	17	8
Heparin	91	85
Dextran infusion	3	-
Leg stockings	55	36
Calf compression	34	3
Electrical stimulation of calves	2	2
Warfarin	7	5
Heel supports	45	4
Ripple mattress	9	3
Other	4	2

Table A30
Time of start of anaesthetic

08:00 to 18:00	213
18:01 to 24:00	52
00:01 to 07:59	15

Table A31
Day of operation

Monday	48
Tuesday	59
Wednesday	45
Thursday	47
Friday	33
Saturday	24
Sunday	22
Bank holiday	2

Table A32
The grade of the most senior <u>surgeon</u> in the operating room

House officer	2
Senior house officer	7
Registrar	57
Staff grade	9
Senior registrar	27
Associate specialist	11
Consultant	165
Not answered	2

Table A33
Was there a trained anaesthetist's assistant present for this case?

Yes   270
No   5
Not answered   5

Table A34
Did the patient receive intravenous fluids during the operation?

Yes   251
No   18
Not answered   11

If yes, which?

Crystalloid

Dextrose 5%   10
Dextrose 4% saline 0.18%   26
Dextrose 10%   3
Saline 0.9%   75
Hartmann's   165
Other   11
None   21

Colloid (and others)

Modified gelatin   130
Human albumin solution   12
Starch (HES)   16
Dextran   3
Mannitol   10
Other   6
None   103

Blood

Whole blood   40
Platelets   8
Fresh frozen plasma   15
Other component   37
None   173

Table A35
Were monitoring devices used during the management of this anaesthetic?

Yes   280

If yes, which?

	Anaesthetic room	Operating room
Room not used	83	6
ECG	174	270
Pulse oximeter	196	274
Indirect BP	158	223
Pulse meter	42	71
Oesophageal or precordial (chest wall) stethoscope	4	8
Fresh gas O_2 analyser	44	170
Inspired gas O_2 analyser	46	221
Inspired anaesthetic vapour analyser	20	183
Expired CO_2 analyser	47	240
Airway pressure gauge	39	212
Ventilation volume	25	183
Ventilation disconnect device	31	209
Peripheral nerve stimulator	6	68
Temperature	8	54
Urine output	21	141
CVP	22	107
Direct arterial BP (invasive)	22	85
Pulmonary arterial pressure	2	22
Intracranial pressure	-	3
Electro-encephalogram/cerebral function analysing monitor/evoked responses	-	-
Other	1	7

Deaths (anaesthetic questionnaires)   100

Table A36
Type of anaesthetic

General alone	210
Regional alone	11
General and regional	30
General and local infiltration	10
Sedation alone	3
Sedation and local infiltration	5
Sedation and regional	11

GENERAL ANAESTHESIA (total number of cases = 250)

Table A37
Did you take precautions at induction to minimise pulmonary aspiration?

Yes	124
No	81
Not answered	5

If yes, which?

Cricoid pressure	84
Postural changes - head up	7
Postural changes - head down	1
Postural changes - lateral	1
Preoxygenation without inflation of lungs	96
Aspiration of nasogastric tube	31
Trachea already intubated on arrival in theatre	30
Other	8

Table A38
How was the airway established during anaesthesia?

Face mask (with or without oral airway)	7
Laryngeal mask	25
Orotracheal intubation	194
Nasotracheal intubation	2
Endobronchial	5
Tracheostomy	1
Patient already intubated prior to arrival in theatre suite	19
Other	4
Not answered	1

Table A39
If the trachea was intubated, how was the position of the tube confirmed?

Tube seen passing through cords	166
Chest movement with inflation	176
Auscultation	132
Expired CO_2 monitoring	166
Other	6

Table A40
Were there any problems with airway maintenance or ventilation?

Yes	7
No	237
Not answered	6

REGIONAL ANAESTHESIA

Table A41
If the anaesthetic included a regional technique, which method was used?

Epidural - caudal	1
Epidural - lumbar	2
Subarachnoid (spinal)	19

Table A42
Which agent was used?

Local	21
Narcotic	2
Other	2

Table A43 (regional only)
Was oxygen given?

Yes	22

If yes, why?

Routine	18
Otherwise indicated	6

SEDATION

Table A44
Which sedative drugs were given for this procedure?

Inhalant	1
Narcotic analgesic	5
Benzodiazepine	5
Sub-anaesthetic doses of IV anaesthetic drugs	2

Table A45 (sedation only)
Was oxygen given?

Yes	8

If yes, why?

Routine	7
Otherwise indicated	2

ALL CASES

Table A46
Where did this patient go on leaving theatre?

Recovery area or room equipped and staffed to this purpose	176
High dependency unit (HDU)	6
Intensive care unit (IDU)	61
Specialised ICU	20
Ward	3
Other	1
Died in theatre	10
Not answered	3

Table A47
Would this destination for patients represent your normal practice after this procedure?

Total number of cases = 270 (excludes patients who died in theatre).

Yes	195
No	30
Not answered	45

Table A48
Were you at any time unable to transfer the patient into ICU/HDU, etc?

Yes	14
No	219
Not answered	47

If yes, why?

Lack of beds	8
No ICU or HDU in hospital	4
Other	2

PATIENTS WHO ENTERED THE RECOVERY ROOM

(Total number = 176)

Table A49
Were monitoring devices used, or investigations carried out, during the management of this patient in the recovery room?

Yes	170
No	1
Not answered	5

If yes, which monitors?

ECG	105
Pulse oximeter	169
Indirect BP	163
Pulse meter	28
Inspired gas O_2 analyser	1
Expired CO_2 analyser	1
Airway pressure gauge	1
Ventilation volume	2
Ventilator disconnect device	2
Temperature	21
Urine output	42
CVP	23
Direct arterial BP (invasive)	4
Blood gas analysis	4
Other	3

Table A50
Where did this patient go next (i.e. after the recovery room)?

Ward	153
High dependency unit (HDU)	15
Intensive care unit (ICU)	5
Specialised ICU	2
Not answered	1

Deaths (anaesthetic questionnaires)

103

Table A51
Was controlled ventilation used postoperatively?

(Total = 270, excludes those who died in theatre)

Yes	83
No	181
Not answered	6

If yes, why? (answers may be multiple)

Routine management	25
Respiratory inadequacy	27
Cardiac inadequacy	17
Control of intracranial pressure or other neurosurgical indications	1
Part of the management of pain	3
Poor general condition of the patient	18
To allow recovery of body temperature	8

Table A52
Did any of the following events, which required specific treatment, occur during anaesthesia or immediate recovery (i.e. the first few hours after the end of the operation)?

Yes	87
No	183
Not answered	10

If yes, specific events:

Air embolus	2
Airway obstruction	1
Anaphylaxis	1
Arrhythmia	17
Bradycardia (to or less than 50% of resting)	9
Bronchospasm	4
Cardiac arrest (unintended)	15
Hypertension (increase of more than 50% resting systolic)	6
Hypotension (decrease of more than 50% resting systolic)	51
Hypoxaemia	9
Misplaced tracheal tube	1
Pulmonary aspiration	2
Pulmonary oedema	3
Tachycardia (increase of 50% or more)	8
Unintentional delayed recovery of consciousness	4
Ventilatory inadequacy	11
Other	9

Table A53
What were the complications or events after this operation?

Ventilatory problems	106
Cardiac problems	102
Hepatic failure	12
Septicaemia	62
Renal failure	61
Central nervous system failure	27
Progress of surgical condition	46
Electrolyte imbalance	21
Haematological disorder/coagulopathy	36
Other	38
Not answered	53

Table A54
Were drugs given in the first 48 hours after operation for pain?

Total = 270 (excludes deaths in theatre)

Yes	238
No	21
Not answered	11

If yes, which drug type?

Opiate/opioid	207
Local analgesic	23
Non-steroidal analgesic	33
Other	22
Not answered	2

If yes, by which method/route?

Intra-muscular injection	83
Oral	60
Rectal	9
Continuous intravenous infusion	76
Patient-controlled analgesia	28
Continuous epidural	20
Patient-controlled epidural analgesia	2
Inhaled	1
Other	11
Not answered	1

Table A55
Did complications occur as a result of these analgesic methods?

(Total = 238)

Yes	4
No	233
Not answered	1

Table A56
Were other sedative/hypnotic or other drugs given?

Yes	93
No	157
Not answered	20

If yes, which?

Propofol	44
Midazolam	38
Other benzodiazepine	6
Other	17

Table A57
Number of calendar days from operation to death

Day of operation	21
One	27
Two	23
Three	11
Four	14
Five	9
Six	12
Seven	10
Eight	8
Nine	14
Ten	8
Eleven to fifteen	41
Sixteen to twenty	33
Twenty-one to twenty-five	23
Twenty-six to thirty	26

Table A58
Place of death

Theatre	11
Intensive care unit	88
High dependency unit	10
Ward	136
Home	13
Another hospital	10
Other	11

Table A59
Do you have morbidity/mortality review meetings in your department?

Yes	259
No	21

If yes, will this case be, or has it been discussed at your departmental meeting?

Yes	74
No	181
Not answered	4

Review of the deaths (surgical questionnaires)

During the year 1995-96 local reporters informed NCEPOD of 19,841 deaths occurring in hospital within 30 days of the patient's final operation. This figure remains remarkably constant from year to year and the regional breakdown is given in appendix F.

A separate group of patients was identified where death occurred following an operation which was within our sample looking at times of surgery; there were 508 deaths in this group. For 473 of the patients in this latter group a surgical questionnaire was sent to the consultant surgeon/gynaecologist in charge of the case. Three hundred and ten questionnaires were returned, a return rate of 65.5% (310/473).

The reports of the other 35 cases were received too late to send questionnaires.

The age and sex distribution of the patients was as expected with a preponderance of patients over 60 years of age and an equal number of men and women. Seventy-one percent (221/310) were urgent or emergency admissions and 72% (224/310) of patients were classed as ASA 3 or higher; 82% (253/310) suffered from at least one coexisting disease, of which cardiorespiratory disease was the most common followed by malignancy (table S13). Most deaths followed general surgical or orthopaedic procedures (S10), 58% (181/310) of the operations were urgent or emergencies (S18) and surgeons stated that 51% (157/310) of these operations carried a definite risk for the patient (S16). These figures are very similar to other NCEPOD studies of larger samples.

The authors and advisors were concerned about the lack of preoperative preparation received by many of these patients who died; particular attention is drawn to the low use of intravenous fluids, infrequent use of objective cardiac assessment and patchy application of thromboembolic prophylaxis.

A consultant was the most senior surgeon in 173 operations and there was senior supervision in a further 51 cases (S21/22). Thus senior surgeons were involved in the surgery of 224 out of 310 (72%) patients who died after surgery. It should be remembered that most of these patients were seriously ill and undergoing urgent/emergency surgery. It is noticeable that 76 of these patients were operated on by senior house officers or registrars. The most common postoperative complications were cardiorespiratory, renal failure and nutritional problems (S26) and there were few difficulties with availability of, or admission to, critical areas such as intensive care of higher dependency units.

Audit remains a partially effective tool for clinical practice; 24% (74/310) of these deaths were not considered at a local quality/audit meeting. It is also of concern that difficulties in obtaining the notes of deceased patients were reported in 14% (42/310) of questionnaires; a constant problem highlighted in previous NCEPOD reports.

With regard to individual patients, the authors and advisory groups identified several themes concerning suboptimal standards of delivery of care. These mainly concerned delays in admission and surgery, inappropriate grades of surgeon (too junior), failure of preoperative preparation, lack of communication between specialties and inappropriate operations. These problems have all been identified in previous NCEPOD reports and recommendations made repetitively.

The thrust of this current study was to analyse the pattern of work within our operating theatres and there is little to be gained by further discussion of this small number of deaths.

Deaths (surgical questionnaires)

Total number = 310

Table S1
In which type of hospital did this operation take place?

District General (or equivalent)	202
University/teaching	93
Surgical specialty	11
Other acute/partly acute	3
Independent	1

Table S2
Are the following areas available in the hospital in which the operation took place?

Theatre recovery area

Yes	309
Not answered	1

If yes, is this available and staffed 24 hours per day, 7 days per week?

Yes	217
No	70
Not answered	22

Adult ICU

Yes	300
No	9
Not answered	1

If yes, is this available and staffed 24 hours per day, 7 days per week?

Yes	273
No	1
Not answered	26

Adult HDU

Yes	145
No	159
Not answered	6

If yes, is this available and staffed 24 hours per day, 7 days per week?

Yes	112
No	11
Not answered	22

Table S3
Age of the patient at the time of this operation

0 to 10	3
11 to 20	2
21 to 30	3
31 to 40	4
41 to 50	11
51 to 60	23
61 to 70	78
71 to 80	98
81 to 90	74
over 90	14

Table S4
Sex of the patient

Male	167
Female	143

Table S5
Admission category

Elective	89
Urgent	27
Emergency	194

Table S6
What was the pathway for this admission?

Transfer as an inpatient from another hospital	26
Transfer from other non-surgical hospital, nursing home etc.	12
Referral from a General Medical Practitioner	111
Admission following a previous outpatient consultation	64
Admission via A & E department	69
Other	27
Not answered	1

Table S7
Type of referring hospital (transferred in patients only)

Total number = 26

District General	17
University/teaching	8
Independent	1

Table S8
To what type of area was the patient first admitted in the hospital in which the operation took place?

Surgical ward (including surgical specialties)	208
Gynaecological/obstetric ward	5
Medical ward	32
Mixed medical/surgical ward	7
Geriatric ward	11
Admission ward	7
A & E holding area/emergency admission ward	11
Day unit	3
Direct to theatre	10
Intensive care unit	5
Coronary care unit	4
High dependency unit	2
Other	5

Table S9
Was there any delay in either the referral or the admission of this patient?

Yes	34
No	257
Not answered	19

Table S10
Specialty of consultant surgeon in charge at the time of this operation

General	25
General with special interest in paediatric surgery	1
General with special interest in urology	7
General with special interest in vascular surgery	48
General with special interest in gastroenterology	53
General with special interest in gastroenterology and endocrinology	6
General with special interest (other)	24
Vascular	9
Urology	24
Transplantation	1
Cardiac/thoracic/cardiothoracic	24
Gynaecology	4
Neurosurgery	11
Ophthalmic	6
Oral/maxillofacial	2
Orthopaedic	50
Otorhinolaryngology	7
Paediatric	1
Plastic	3
Other	4

Deaths (surgical questionnaires)

Table S11
What was the grade of the most senior surgeon <u>consulted</u> before the operation?

Senior house officer	3
Registrar	12
Senior registrar	15
Associate specialist	5
Consultant	274
Other	1

Two of the senior registrars and seven of the consultants were locums.

Table S12
ASA class

1	9
2	66
3	117
4	93
5	14
Not answered	11

Table S13
Were there any coexisting problems (other than the main diagnosis) at the time of this operation?

Yes	253
No	47
Not answered	10

If yes, which problems?

Malignancy	46
Respiratory	100
Cardiac	133
Renal	40
Haematological	25
Gastrointestinal	31
Vascular	34
Sepsis	32
Neurological	34
Diabetes mellitus	26
Other endocrine	4
Musculoskeletal	16
Psychiatric	12
Alcohol-related problems	7
Genetic abnormality	1
Other	26

Table S14
What precautions or therapeutic manoeuvres were undertaken preoperatively (excluding anaesthetic room management) to improve the patient's preoperative condition?

None	42
Cardiac support drugs or antidysrhythmic agents	64
Gastric aspiration	74
Intravenous fluids	171
Correction of hypovolaemia	100
Urinary catheterisation	124
Blood transfusion	45
Diuretics	35
Anticoagulants	48
Vitamin K	10
Antibiotics (pre- or intraoperative)	162
Bowel preparation	22
Chest physiotherapy	47
Oxygen therapy	80
Airway protection	18
Tracheal intubation	29
Mechanical ventilation	21
Nutritional support	22
Others	30
Not answered	10

Table S15
Were any measures taken to prevent venous thromboembolism?

Yes   218
No   89
Not answered   3

If yes, methods:

	Before/during	After
Heparin	138	99
Leg stockings	123	90
Calf compression	47	5
Electrical compression of calves	1	1
Warfarin	7	6
Dextran infusion	2	1
Heel support	44	11
Ripple mattress	11	15
Other	5	6
Nil	11	74
Not answered	1	1

Table S16
What was the anticipated risk of death related to the proposed operation?

Not expected   72
Small but significant risk 78
Definite risk   135
Expected   22
Not answered   3

Table S17
Were there any delays (between admission and surgery) due to factors other than clinical?

Yes   25
No   283
Not answered   2

Table S18
Classification of the operation

Emergency   47
Urgent   134
Scheduled   91
Elective   38

Table S19
Time of start of operation

	Weekday	Saturday	Sunday
08.00 to 18.00	212	14	14
18.01 to 23.59	41	10	3
24.00 to 07.59	11	2	3

Table S20
Which grades of surgeon were present in the operating room during the procedure?

House officer   13
Senior house officer   123
Registrar   129
Staff grade   16
Senior registrar   58
Clinical assistant   4
Associate specialist   13
Consultant   195
Other   2
Not answered   5

In three cases, two consultants were present. These figures include locums - two SHOs, four registrars, four senior registrars, one associate specialist and four consultants.

Table S21
What was the grade of the most senior operating surgeon?

Senior house officer (SHO)	11
Registrar	65
Staff grade	11
Senior registrar	37
Clinical assistant	2
Associate specialist	11
Consultant	173

These figures include locums - three registrars, four senior registrars, one associate specialist and four consultants.

Table S22
If the most senior operator was not a consultant, was a more senior surgeon immediately available, i.e. in the operating room/suite?

Yes	51
No	77
Not answered	9

Table S23
Were there any unanticipated intra-operative problems?

Yes	39
No	267
Not answered	4

Table S24
Was the patient admitted to an ICU or HDU immediately after leaving the theatre suite?

Intensive care unit (ICU)	91
High dependency unit (HDU)	24
Neither of the above	184
Died on table	5
Not answered	6

If neither, was the patient admitted to an ICU/HDU after an initial period on a routine postoperative ward?

Intensive care unit (ICU)	18
High dependency unit (HDU)	3
Neither of the above	156
Not answered	7

Table S25
Discharge from ICU/HDU was due to:

(Total = 136)

Death	96
Elective transfer to ward	31
Pressure on beds	1
Other	5
Not answered	3

Table S26
Postoperative complications

(Total cases = 305, excludes deaths on table)

Haemorrhage/postoperative bleeding requiring transfusion	26
Upper respiratory obstruction	8
Respiratory distress	83
Generalised sepsis	48
Wound infection/dehiscence	18
Anastomotic failure	8
Cardiac arrest	53
Low cardiac output/other cardiac problems	90
Hepatic failure	13
Renal failure	48
Endocrine system failure	2
Stroke or other neurological problems	12
Persistent coma	6
Other organ failure	9
Problems with analgesia	1
Deep vein thrombosis	4
Pulmonary embolus	9
Orthopaedic prosthetic complication	2
Pressure sores	3
Peripheral ischaemia	9
Urinary tract infection	6
Urinary retention/catheter blockage	3
Nutritional problems	17
Other	42
None	37
Not answered	13

Table S27
Was there a shortage of personnel in this case?

Yes	5
No	294
Not answered	11

Table S28
Calendar days from operation to death

Day of operation	26
One	25
Two	20
Three	17
Four	15
Five	12
Six	13
Seven	6
Eight	9
Nine	14
Ten	6
Eleven to fifteen	48
Sixteen to twenty	39
Twenty-one to twenty-five	30
Twenty-six to thirty	30

Table S29
Place of death

Theatre	9
Recovery room	2
Ward	157
ICU/HDU	104
Coronary care unit	2
Home	14
Another acute hospital	5
Other	14
Not known	1
Not answered	2

Table S30
Has this death been considered (or will it be considered) at a local audit/quality control meeting?

Yes	217
No	74
Not answered	19

Table S31
Did you have any problems in obtaining the patient's notes (i.e. more than one week)?

Yes	42
No	255
Not answered	13

Table S32
Were all the notes available?

Yes	247
No	48
Not answered	15

If no, which part was inadequate/unavailable?

Preoperative notes	1
Operative notes	6
Postoperative notes	5
Death certificate book	24
Nursing notes	5
Anaesthetic notes	9
Postmortem report	12
Other notes	8
Not answered	3

Appendices

APPENDIX A

Participating NHS Trusts (number of hospitals) and independent sector hospitals, with names of local coordinators (*) and providers of data.

Anglia & Oxford

Addenbrooke's	(1)	J. McArdle*
Bedford Hospitals	(1)	D J Niblett*
Royal Berkshire & Battle Hospitals	(2)	S Kearns* , V Tuthill
Heatherwood & Wexham Park Hospitals	(1)	P J Hatton*, W A P McDowell
Hinchingbrooke	(1)	M R Dadds*
Horton General Hospital	(1)	M T Brunker, J A Orr*
Ipswich Hospital	(1)	I H K Scott*, M Winter
Kings Lynn & Wisbech	(2)	M D Cairns, Y M Eastgate, M L Reason, C Weston*
(Queen Elizabeth Hospital, North Cambridgeshire Hospital)		
Luton & Dunstable Hospital	(1)	M V L Foss, K Golts, L A Jones, K Mandaleson*, P S Weir
Milton Keynes General Hospital	(1)	P T Dilworth*
Norfolk & Norwich Hospital	(4)	C Dodd*
(Norfolk and Norwich Hospital, West Norwich Hospital		
Cromer and District Hospital, St Michael's Hospital)		
Nuffield Orthopaedic Centre	(1)	J Chalmers*, M Haynes
Papworth Hospital	(1)	R D Gill, S Nashef*, J Younger
Peterborough Hospitals	(2)	N Dawkins*, D Healy, C B Lutkin
(Peterborough District Hospital, Edith Cavell Hospital)		
The Radcliffe Infirmary	(1)	J Chalmers, O Senior*
Stoke Mandeville Hospital	(1)	R D Atfield*
West Suffolk Hospitals	(1)	S L Campey, L Earp, S Smith*

North Thames

St Albans and Hemel Hempstead	(2)	S Hill*, K P Hilton, S Townsend, V Townsend
Basildon & Thurrock General Hospitals	(2)	J Galpin, S Jennings*, A Whittle
(Basildon Hospital, Orsett Hospital)		
Chase Farm Hospitals	(1)	K Hanlon*
Chelsea & Westminster Healthcare	(1)	D Highton*, M Sampson
Central Middlesex	(1)	J F Riordan*, J Silkoff
Ealing Hospital	(1)	R Donovan, J Howe, C Schmulian*
East Hertfordshire Health	(2)	A Cooke, P A Rogers*
(Hertford County Hospital, Queen Elizabeth II Hospital)		

Appendix A (participating hospitals)

North Thames continued

Forest Healthcare	(1)	B P Andrews*, N Clarke, J Davidson, J E Stott
(Whipps Cross Hospital)		
Great Ormond Street Hospital	(1)	S Dutch
Hammersmith & Charing Cross	(3)	F M Kergoat*, R Lacey, A M Thomson, P Yelland
(Hammersmith Hospital, Charing Cross Hospital, Queen Charlotte's and Chelsea Hospital)		
Harefield Hospital	(1)	K Boston*
Hillingdon Hospital	(1)	S Barrington*, R Stephenson
Homerton Hospital	(1)	E Farragher*
Mid-Essex Hospital Services	(3)	J Ardley*, P Dines*, R A Spilsbury
Black Notley Hospital, Broomfield Hospital, St John's Hospital)		
Moorfields Eye Hospital	(1)	R A Hitchings*
Mount Vernon & Watford Hospitals	(2)	J Jones*
The National Hospital for Neurology and Neurosurgery	(1)	M H Browne, A Jackson*
North Herts	(1)	D Griffiths*, J Kilminster
(Lister Hospital)		
North Middlesex Hospital	(1)	T Dey, L Pibworth*
Northwick Park & St Mark's Hospitals	(1)	R J Nicholls*, C Speakman, C J Vaizey
(St Mark's Hospital)		
The Princess Alexandra Hospital	(3)	L Hardstaff*, S Skingsley
(Herts and Essex General Hospital, Princess Alexandra Hospital, St Margaret's Hospital)		
Redbridge Healthcare	(1)	I Mackay*, C Miles
(King George Hospital)		
Royal Free Hampstead	(1)	J Sigsworth*, L J Stephens
The Royal Hospitals	(3)	S Lane*, J McMurdie
(London Chest Hospital, The Royal London Hospital, St Bartholomew's Hospital)		
The Royal Marsden Hospital	(2)	R J Shearer*
Royal National Orthopaedic Hospital	(1)	N Daniel, J Robinson*, J Rodney
Royal National Throat, Nose & Ear Hospital	(1)	L Beck, K C Maduako*
Southend Healthcare	(2)	C Brand, P Hadfield*, P Unsworth, J Willis
(Rochford Hospital, Southend Hospital)		
University College London Hospitals	(3)	C Hornick, S Knowles*
(Elizabeth Garret Anderson Hospital, Middlesex Hospital, University College Hospital)		
Wellhouse	(2)	N Beverley*, T M Murphy
(Barnet General Hospital, Edgware General Hospital)		
Whittington Hospital	(1)	A Johnson, N Parker*

Appendix A (participating hospitals)

North West

Aintree Hospitals
(Walton Hospital, Fazakerley Hospital) — (2) — S Bajaj*, A Peate

Blackburn, Hyndburn & Ribble Valley
(Blackburn Royal Infirmary, Queen's Park Hospital) — (2) — M Spotswood*

Bolton Hospitals
(Royal Bolton Hospital, Bolton Royal Infirmary) — (2) — S A Fox*

Blackpool Victoria Hospital
(Blackpool Victoria Hospital, Fleetwood Hospital, Lytham St Anne's Hospital, South Shore Hospital) — (4) — V Woodcock*

Burnley Health Care
(Burnley General Hospital, Rossendale General Hospital) — (2) — S J Frizelle, M G Pratt*

Bury Health Care
(Bury General Hospital, Fairfield General Hospital) — (2) — B Lynch, J Mackenzie, E Meredith*, D Partington, K Ryan

Cardiothoracic Centre - Liverpool — (1) — M Jackson

Countess of Chester Hospital — (1) — F Morland*, P R M Steele*

East Cheshire
(Macclesfield District General Hospital) — (1) — N Ambage*, D Johnson, A J Kirk,

Furness Hospitals — (1) — K Quigley*, L Twomey

Halton General Hospital — (1) — C B Sellars*, H Wilcockson

Lancaster Acute Hospitals
(Royal Lancaster Infirmary, Lancaster Moor Hospital) — (2) — G Hind*, C M Tite

Liverpool Women's Hospital NHS Trust — (1) — A Burn*, M G Dunn

Manchester Central Hospitals
(Manchester Royal Infirmary, St Mary's Hospital, Manchester Royal Eye Hospital, Turner Dental School) — (4) — J M Grabham, J M Thomas, D Woodyatt*

North Manchester Healthcare — (1) — D Coggins, H Mullen*, D Young

Preston Acute Hospitals
(Sharoe Green Hospital, Royal Preston Hospital) — (2) — D Hudson*, S Pay

Royal Liverpool Children's Hospital — (1) — L Hannam*, P A McCormack, C S Smith

Royal Liverpool University Hospital — (1) — A Cogan, J Lawes*

Royal Manchester Children's Hospital
(Royal Manchester Children's Hospital, Booth Hall Children's Hospital) — (2) — T Hardcastle, M McDermott, F Murphy*

Rochdale Health Care
(Birch Hill Hospital, Rochdale Infirmary) — (2) — C Flatt, S A Murray*

Royal Oldham Hospital — (1) — G Oates, S Taylor, M Tomlinson*

Appendix A (participating hospitals)

North West continued

St Helens & Knowsley
(Whiston Hospital, St Helen's Hospital) — C J Sanderson* (2)

Salford Hospitals
(Hope Hospital) — E M Craddock*, M McKenna (1)

South Manchester University Hospitals
(University Hospital of South Manchester, Wythenshawe Hospital, Duchess of York Children's Hospital) — C M H Brown*, M Leyland, E M Sneyd (3)

Stockport Acute Services
(Stepping Hill Hospital, Stockport Infirmary) — E Donegan*, M Gillespie, P J Patterson (2)

Tameside & Glossop Acute Services — J R Butterworth, A S Day, A Ingham, M Stevens (1)

Walton Centre for Neurology and Neurosurgery — S D Harrison* (1)

Warrington Acute — C M Reed* (1)

Wigan & Leigh Health Services
(Royal Albert Edward Infirmary, Billinge Hospital, Leigh Infirmary) — I Gupta*, S E Tarbuck (3)

West Lancashire
(Ormskirk & District General Hospital) — S Fishwick, R G Hammond* (1)

Westmorland Hospitals — E McCall* (1)

Wrightington Hospital — V Abernethy*, J Clarke (1)

Northern and Yorkshire

Airedale — S Crane*, C Riley (1)

Bishop Auckland Hospitals — R Wansborough* (1)

Calderdale Healthcare
(Halifax General Hospital, Royal Halifax Infirmary) — D Connolly, A Gee*, L Throp (2)

Carlisle Hospitals
(City General Hospital, Cumberland Infirmary) — D F Jones, P Wiggins* (2)

Cheviot & Wansbeck
(Wansbeck General Hospital, Ashington Hospital) — J Pledger* (2)

Darlington Memorial Hospital — M Conner, C Evans*, L Stewart (1)

Dewsbury Health Care — E M Faulkner, S Midgley* (1)

North East Lincolnshire
(Grimsby District General Hospital) — C Davies*, K Lee, W M Peters (1)

Harrogate Health
(Harrogate District Hospital, Harrogate General Hospital) — A H Lawson* (2)

Huddersfield — L McBride*, Y Roberts (1)

Northallerton Health Services — A Thomas, M R Walton* (1)

North Tees Health — P Warwick, S Pearce* (1)

Appendix A (participating hospitals)

Northern & Yorkshire continued

North Tyneside Health Care — J E Black, C Gibson*, E C Gibson, (1)

Pinderfields Hospital — M E Dodgson, R L Ladley, G Macdonald*, A Walker (2)
(Clayton Hospital, Pinderfields General Hospital)

Pontefract Hospitals — P T Donnelly*, E Thornley (1)

Royal Victoria Infirmary Group — I Anderson, R A L Brewis*, S Cook, L A Donnelly, J P Forsey (3)
(Newcastle General Hospital, Royal Victoria Infirmary, Hexham General Hospital)

Scunthorpe & Goole Hospitals — S Conroy, J Doyle, M McCormick* (2)
(Scunthorpe General Hospital, Goole and District Hospital)

St James's & Seacroft University Hospitals — J Sleight* (2)

South Tees Acute Hospitals — P Osbourne* (3)
(Middlesbrough General Hospital, North Riding Infirmary, South Cleveland Hospital)

South Tyneside Health Care — D Campbell, E B Denyer, P Donoghue, D Shilton* (1)

United Leeds Teaching Hospitals — S Ambler, P Bijsterveld, I Brown, P Clark, A M Colquhoun, S J Craven, M Jakeways, S Nixon, H O'Donnell*, M Rutherford, J Towers, S Ward (5)
(Killingbeck Hospital, Chapel Allerton Hospital, Leeds General Infirmary, Leeds Dental Institute, Wharfedale General Hospital)

West Cumbria Health Care — F Armstrong, M Hartley* (1)

York Health Services — C A Jenvey, G Sheath* (1)

South Thames

Ashford Hospital — N Devonport, G Mynors, M van Limborgh* (1)

Bromley Hospitals — D J McCormack* (3)
(Bromley Hospital, Farnborough Hospital, Orpington Hospital)

Crawley & Horsham — A Burrage*, V Harding (2)

Dartford & Gravesham — F Annea, R J C Evans*, W Siveyer (3)
(Gravesend & North Kent Hospital, Joyce Green Hospital, West Hill Hospital)

Eastbourne Hospitals — M D Bastable*, C S Nevin, D Stent, M Underwood (1)

Epsom Health Care — K Hider* (1)

East Surrey Hospital — L Candwell, S Shaylor*, C D White (1)

Frimley Park Hospital — V Cook*, A Ince, K Matthews (1)

Greenwich Healthcare — P Cook, J de Bene*, C Swift, V Turkington, S L Turner (3)
(Brook General Hospital, Greenwich District Hospital, Queen Elizabeth Military Hospital)

Guy's & St Thomas' — D Bolton, C Cranston, V Dutchin, T J Matthews, J Parkes* (2)

Hastings & Rother — M Basden*, S Holmes S J Hopkins, A Moller, E A Sturt (3)
(Bexhill Hospital, Buchanan Hospital, Conquest Hospital)

Appendix A (participating hospitals)

St Helier — J S Catling*, V M Lipscombe — (4)
(Nelson Hospital, Queen Mary's Hospital for Children, St Helier Hospital, Sutton Hospital)

Kent & Canterbury Hospitals — G Prescott*, D Watts — (1)

King's Healthcare — A P Fisher* — (1)

Kingston Hospital — K Lyons, T Tillin* — (1)

The Medway — P A Baker, H Belcher*, D J Dawson, J K Henderson, S Humphrey, J M Levy, S C S Potter, N Read, C D Stephens, D Wigley — (3)
(All Saints' Hospital, Medway Hospital, St Bartholomew's Hospital)

Mid-Kent Healthcare — N Jones* — (2)
(Kent County Ophthalmic & Aural Hospital, The Maidstone Hospital)

Mid-Sussex — H Adams, A Crawford, D Goodger*, S A Marsden, C Pye — (2)
(Hurstwood Park Neurology Centre, Princess Royal Hospital) — S Thomas*, P H Walter

St Peter's Hospital — CA Fahy*, R H Moore — (1)

Queen Mary's Sidcup — M Bassilious, J Millard* — (1)

The Royal West Sussex — E Tuke* — (1)

South Kent Hospitals — J M Killick, S Turbutt* — (3)
(Buckland Hospital, William Harvey Hospital, Victoria Hospital)

St George's Health Care — G Abdu, S Ashworth, J McCabe* — (2)
(Atkinson Morley's Hospital, St George's Hospital)

Thanet Health Care — A Kindred*, L Nicholls, H J Wilton — (1)
(Queen Elizabeth the Queen Mother Hospital)

Worthing & Southlands Hospital — I M Jackson, G North* — (2)

South West

East Gloucestershire — W J Brampton* — (4)
(Cheltenham General Hospital, St Paul's Hospital, Cirencester Memorial Hospital, Tewkesbury Hospital)

East Somerset (Yeovil District Hospital) — M Burridge*, Y Thorne — (1)

Frenchay Health Care — J Hopes, A Lloyd* — (1)

Gloucestershire Royal — T Tomlinson*, J Wells — (1)

Northern Devon Health Care — W P Bradford*, R Lilley, B S Sheppard — (1)

Plymouth Hospitals — C G Taylor* — (3)
(Plymouth General Hospital, Derriford Hospital, The Royal Eye Infirmary)

Poole Hospital — J K Myatt* — (1)

Portsmouth Hospitals — E Cooper, J L Crawford, W D Flatman, H Newberry, N J Webb, J R B Young — (2)
(St Mary's Hospital, Queen Alexandra Hospital)

Appendix A (participating hospitals)

South West continued

Royal United Hospital Bath — C J Chapman* (1)

Royal Cornwall Hospitals — C Beaman, J Freeman* (3)
(Royal Cornwall Hospital, Falmouth & District Hospital, West Corwall Hospital)

St Mary's Hospital (Isle of Wight Acute) — P Grimaldi*, I J F Morle, C Willis (1)

Salisbury Health Care — C Perren, M Smith* (1)

South Devon Healthcare — R F Neale*, J L Thorn (4)
(Torbay Hospital, Newton Abbot Hospital, Paignton Hospital, Teignmouth Hospital)

Southmead Hospital — I Dawson, C J H Johnson* (1)

Southampton University Hospitals — N Barlow, N Baverstock, C A Foster, R Grant*, E R Long, Y Morrison, J Sansome, G P Tyler (4)
(Southampton General Hospital, Princess Anne Hospital, Royal South Hants Hospital, Southampton Eye Hospital)

Swindon & Marlborough — I Ausejs, V E A Culpeper*, J Lamonby (3)
(Princess Margaret Hospital, Savernake Hospital, Princess Alexandra's RAF Hospital)

Taunton & Somerset — S M Jones* (1)

West Dorset General Hospitals — N J Chapman, M Hill, I A Jenkins*, R Samways, P Somani (3)
(Dorset County Hospital, West Dorset General Hospital, Weymouth & District Hospital)

Winchester & Eastleigh Healthcare — G J Boyle, S Dailly, S Davis, J Robson* (1)
Royal Hampshire County Hospital)

Trent

Barnsley District General Hospital — S Collins*, S Williamson (1)

Bassetlaw Hospital — S Green, D McCammick*, C Tattersall (1)

Chesterfield & North Derbyshire Royal — I R Gell* (1)

Central Sheffield University Hospitals — J Chapman*, G Firkins (2)
(Jessop Hospital for Women, Royal Hallamshire Hospital)

Derby City General Hospital — K Hillier-Smith, E Lycitt*, S Mayne, R H Smith (1)

Derbyshire Royal Infirmary — J M Turton* (2)
(Derbyshire Royal Infirmary, Bretby Hall Orthopaedic Hospital)

Doncaster Royal Infirmary — J A H Finbow, Y Walley (2)
(Doncaster Royal Infirmary, Montagu Hospital)

Glenfield Hospital — S Lee, E Simons* (1)

Leicester General Hospital — W W Barrie, S J Lamont (1)

Leicester Royal Infirmary — J House, D F Watkin* (1)

Appendix A (participating hospitals)

Trent continued

Lincoln Hospitals (2) A M Bishop, K Charles, J Evans, S E Gray, J Stonham*
(Lincoln County Hospital, St George's Hospital)

Louth & District Healthcare (1) J C Burke*, L W Hecht

Nottingham City Hospital (1) N G Nice*

Northern General Hospital (1) J E Clewes, J Moore*

Pilgrim Health (1) C Holliday*, C J Raliman

Queen's Medical Centre, Nottingham (1) P Kemp*, J Scott

Rotherham General Hospitals (1) H Gooch*, S Hayball

Sheffield Children's Hospital (1) I Barker*

West Lindsey (1) P Byron, J Gyles, A Procter*
(John Coupland Hospital)

West Midlands

Alexandra Healthcare (1) C Davis*, B Smith, S Steer

Birmingham Children's Hospital (1) C Hough*, J Stickley

Birmingham Heartlands Hospital (2) P J Milligan, M Taylor*, M Wilson*
(Birmingham Heartlands Hospital, Solihull Hospital)

Burton Hospitals (2) P M Hobbs, M Hughes*
(Burton General Hospital, Burton District Hospital Centre)

City Hospitals (2) R Kay*
(Dudley Road Hospital, Birmingham & Midland Eye Hospital)

Dudley Group of Hospitals (4) G Biersa, R J Blunt*
(Guest Hospital, Russells Hall Hospital, Wordsley Hospital, The Corbett Hospital)

The George Eliot Hospital (1) J C Duffy*

Good Hope Hospital (1) J Mason, F P Murray*

Hereford Hospitals (3) S M Probert*, A Sheppard
(The County Hospital, The General Hospital, Victoria Eye Hospital)

Kidderminster Healthcare (1) P Armitstead*, C Martin

North Staffordshire Hospital Centre (3) J C Bridgewater, W F Eggington, S D Gray*, M Hodgson
(North Staffordshire Royal Infirmary, Hartshill Orthopaedic Hospital, The City General Hospital)

The Princess Royal (1) D Christmas*, H Coleman

Robert Jones & Agnes Hunt (1) P M Pfeifer*

Royal Orthopaedic Hospital (1) A Thomas*

Royal Shrewsbury Hospitals (2) M A Liquorish, P Skitt*
(Royal Shrewsbury Hospital, Eye, Ear and Throat Hospital)

Appendix A (participating hospitals)

West Midlands continued

Rugby
(Hospital of St Cross)
R C McBride, R McMahon* (1)

The Royal Wolverhampton Hospitals
(New Cross Hospital, The Royal Hospital, Wolverhampton & Midland Counties Eye Infirmary, The Beynon Centre)
L Graff, A P Thomas, P Venables* (4)

Sandwell Healthcare
C Bromley*, D J Ellis (1)

Birmingham University Hospital
(Queen Elizabeth Hospital, Birmingham General Hospital, Selly Oak Hospital)
S Peak, P Tanner* (3)

South Warwickshire General
G M Rushton (1)

Walsall Hospitals (The Manor Hospital)
P B Carpenter*, M Poston (1)

The Walsgrave Hospitals
(Walsgrave Hospital, Coventry & Warwickshire Hospital)
D Bentley*, C A Bradshaw, M T Carroll, J A Dyde, K E Foreman, G D Giles, L H Kingham, G H Rangoonwala, E A Stevens (2)

Worcester Royal Infirmary
(Worcester Royal Infirmary - Castle Street and Ronkswood branches)
A Parberry*, R Stroud (2)

Northern Ireland

Altnagelvin Hospitals
S Burnside, K Ferris, D Hill* (1)

Armagh & Dungannon DMU
(South Tyrone Hospital)
L Moore* (1)

Belfast City Hospital
K Briggs, A McAfee*, M R McDonald (1)
W S Tweed* (1)

Causeway
(Coleraine Hospital)
D Jeffers, M McCaffrey* (1)

Craigavon Area Hospital Group
P A Bramall, C Douglas, J Simpson*, I Younge (2)

Down Lisburn
(Downe Hospital, Lagan Valley Hospital)
J D R Connolly*, J R Nixon (1)

Green Park
(Musgrave Park Hospital)
M Cushina, U Hurrell, P B McKeever*, P G Loughran* (1)

Mater Hospital
(1)

Newry & Mourne
(Daisy Hill Hospital)
R F Bothwell, W Holmes*, F Robinson* (2)

Sperrin Lakeland
(Erne Hospital, Tyrone County Hospital)
P Beresford, J Gaston*, A T Stewart, M Toner (3)

The Royal Group of Hospitals
(Royal Belfast Hospital for Sick Children, The Royal Victoria Hospital, Royal Maternity Hospital)

Appendix A (participating hospitals)

Northern Ireland continued

United Hospitals Group
(Mid-Ulster Hospital, Whiteabbey Hospital, Antrim Hospital)   (3)   D Currie*, D J Grainger*, P C Pyper*

Ulster, North Down & Ards Hospitals
(Ards Hospital, Ulster Hospital)   (2)   A McCalmont, E McMullan*

Wales

Bridgend & District
(Bridgend General Hospital, Princess of Wales Hospital)   (2)   G E Alford, M H Evans, A Faull*

Carmarthen & District
(West Wales General Hospital)   (1)   M J Griffith*, R S Thomas

Ceredigion & Mid Wales
(Bronglais General Hospital)   (1)   J Pugh Jones*, M Morely, J Roberts

East Glamorgan   (1)   M Jones, G Walker*

Glan Clwyd District General Hospital
(Glan Clwyd Hospital, Abergele Hospital)   (2)   A Bailey, R M Dunshea, I Howard*

Glan Hafren
(Royal Gwent Hospital, St Woolos Hospital)   (2)   C Blackborow, L Davies*, S Russell

Glan-Y-Mor
(Neath General Hospital, Port Talbot & District General Hospital)   (2)   P Griffiths, C Havard, J Nickolds, L Phillips*

Gwynedd Hospitals
(Ysbyty Gwynedd, Llandudno General Hospital)   (2)   C Barton*, N Jarret, P S Roberts

Llandough Hospital   (1)   C Ellis*, N D Groves

Llanelli Dinefwr
(Prince Philip Hospital)   (1)   A J Barnett*, M Isaac, J Williams

North Glamorgan
(Prince Charles Hospital)   (1)   D L Davies*, L Neagle, A Slatter

Morriston Hospital   (1)   K C Vaughton*

Nevill Hall & District   (1)   M J Southerden, R A Williams*

Pembrokeshire
(Withybush General Hospital)   (1)   T J Davies*

Appendix A (participating hospitals)

Wales continued

Powys Health Care   (1)   D A Altmeyer, Y J Jones*
(Breconshire War Memorial Hospital)
Rhondda Health Care   (1)   D Davies, M R John, P V Rowland*, B K Williams
(Porth Hospital)   (1)   M Whitehead*
Swansea
(Singleton Hospital)   (2)   R Hicks*, J McGregor*
University Hospital of Wales
(University Hospital of Wales, Cardiff Royal Infirmary)

INDEPENDENT SECTOR

General Healthcare Group plc   D S Anderson, J Lamont, S Saleh*
The Alexandra Hospital and Healthcare Centre (Cheadle)   C Reilly, A Sayburn*, L H Wicks
The Portland Hospital for Women and Children (London)   S J Ruddy*
The Sloane Hospital (Beckenham)

BUPA Hospitals   C Fisher*, M Priestley, E A Vincent
BUPA Belvedere Hospital (Scarborough)   M Vognsen*
BUPA Cambridge Lea Hospital (Cambridge)   P Border, T Hamblin, H Mundella, M E Vockins
BUPA Dunedin Hospital (Reading)   K P Giove*
BUPA Fylde Coast Hospital (Blackpool)   J May*
BUPA Hospital Bristol   C Davies*
BUPA Hospital Bushey   S B Rycroft, M E Schofield*
BUPA Hospital Elland   K M Wilkinson*
BUPA Hospital Hull and East Riding   C A Jones*, E A Williams
BUPA Hospital Leicester   A Abbassi, E Rallings, C S Skitt*
BUPA Hospital Little Aston (Sutton Coldfield)   M Welch*
BUPA Hospital Norwich   A Satterley*
BUPA North Cheshire Hospital (Warrington)   M T Hall*
BUPA Parkway Hospital (Solihull)   N P Austin*
BUPA Roding Hospital (Ilford)   K Brooks, S A Wood
BUPA South Bank Hospital (Worcester)   E Biddle*
BUPA St Saviour's Hospital (Hythe)   E A Hoare*
BUPA Wellesley Hospital (Southend on Sea)   J E A Killips*
BUPA Murrayfield Hospital (Wirral)

Benenden Hospital   J N D Hibler

APPENDIX B

National Confidential Enquiry into Perioperative Deaths

TIMES OF SURGICAL OPERATIONS

Please complete this sheet for all procedures (any specialty) performed by surgeons or gynaecologists starting between 00.01 hrs and 24.00 hrs (midnight) on (date printed here)

(Hospital name printed here)

1 Name of theatre .... 2 Hospital number of patient ....

3 Date of admission [ ][ ][ ][1][9][9][ ]

4 Sex of patient M [ ]   F [ ]   5 Patient's date of birth [ ][ ][ ][ ][ ][ ][ ]

6 Was this patient operated on as a day-case? Yes [ ]   No [ ]

7 Was this procedure performed:

during a scheduled session? [ ]   outside a scheduled session? [ ]

8 What was the <u>type</u> of operating theatre session?

A   scheduled primarily for theatre cases planned in advance   [ ]

B   scheduled primarily for emergency theatre cases   [ ]

C   unscheduled   [ ]

9 Classification of theatre case   Emergency [ ]   Routine [ ]

10 Time of **start** of theatre case [ ][ ][ ][ ]   11 Time out of theatre [ ][ ][ ][ ]

Please turn over the page

12 Primary diagnosis ....

....

13 Procedure(s) performed or OPCS or Read code ....

....

14 Name of consultant surgeon "in charge" ....

15 Name and grade of the most senior surgeon present during the operation

....

16 Name and grade of the most senior anaesthetist present during the operation

....

17 Name (if available) of consultant anaesthetist responsible for this list/procedure or name of on-call consultant anaesthetist

....

APPENDIX C

NOTES ABOUT COMPLETION OF THE QUESTIONNAIRE
(definitions are given on separate sheets included in this pack)

1. General

   Please complete the questionnaire (<u>or</u> include the data in a print-out from your computer system) for <u>every</u> theatre case (see definitions) on the date specified by NCEPOD. You will be notified of the date at least 14 days in advance.

   Please keep this <u>date</u> as confidential as possible. Inform <u>only</u> those people who need to know in order to obtain the data. It is important that the pattern of operating should not be affected by the fact that NCEPOD will be collecting data.

   All of the data will remain confidential at the NCEPOD office. We will be writing to consultant surgeons about some of the cases.

2. <u>NCEPOD definition of a surgical operation:</u>

   Any procedure carried out <u>by a surgeon or gynaecologist</u>, with or without an anaesthetist, involving local, regional or general anaesthesia or sedation.

   Do **not** include obstetric procedures.

   All other surgical specialties should be included. Endoscopy <u>should</u> be included if performed by a surgeon.

3. <u>Theatres</u>

   Please see the list of definitions. Please include the anaesthetic room as a theatre.

   Please <u>exclude</u> procedures which are performed within the accident and emergency department and procedures performed on a ward or in the outpatient department or on the intensive care or high dependency unit.

   Please <u>include</u> procedures performed in a day case unit or theatre.

4. <u>Date of admission (question 3)</u>

   Please enter the date on which the patient was admitted to the hospital (i.e. on the same site) in which the procedure was performed

5. <u>Definition of a day case (question 6)</u>

   A surgical day case is a patient who is admitted for investigations or operation on a planned non-resident basis (i.e. no overnight stay).

6. <u>During or outside a scheduled session</u> (question 7)

   Please see the list of definitions

7. <u>Type of operating theatre session</u> (question 8)

   Please see the list of definitions

8. <u>Classification of theatre case</u>

   Please see the list of definitions.

9. Time of start of theatre case and time out of theatre

Please see the list of definitions.

PLEASE USE THE 24-HOUR CLOCK. For midnight, please enter "24.00".

10. Primary diagnosis (question 12)

We need to know why this procedure was performed. If the primary diagnosis is not available, please indicate the reason for the operation.

11. Procedure(s) performed

Please provide either the name of the procedure or the OPCS4 procedure code or the Read code.

12. Name of consultant surgeon

This should always be the name of a consultant surgeon or gynaecologist in charge of the team performing the operation.

13. Name and grade of most senior anaesthetist present during the operation

Please note that this will not always be the anaesthetist at the beginning of the procedure. If a more senior anaesthetist goes into the theatre, his or her name and grade should be recorded.

If it is not possible to provide this information, please inform the NCEPOD office (the name of the person to contact is shown on the attached sheet).

14. Name of consultant anaesthetist

If the most senior anaesthetist was not a consultant, please provide the name of the consultant anaesthetist who is nominally responsible for the operating list or the name of the consultant anaesthetist who was on call at the time of the operation. If this information is not available, please write "N/Av".

15. What to do with the completed questionnaires or computer print-out

Please send all of the completed questionnaires to us as soon as possible. It is important that we receive the information quickly as we shall be writing to consultant anaesthetists and surgeons about some of the cases. You will need to keep a record of the information sent to us (see section 16).

Send the questionnaires or print-out to the NCEPOD office in the A4-size business reply envelopes provided by NCEPOD. You do not need to address this to a specific person.

16. Deaths

We need to know which of the patients die (either in hospital or at home) within 30 days of the operation. We will write to you to ask for the name and date of death of these patients.

When the information on the deaths has been sent to NCEPOD you can then destroy any record of all of the information sent to us.

THANK YOU FOR YOUR HELP WITH THE ENQUIRY. YOU WILL RECEIVE A COMPLIMENTARY COPY OF THE PUBLISHED REPORT FOR 1995/96.

Please do not hesitate to contact our office if you need any information or assistance.

Appendix C

APPENDIX D

DEFINITIONS*

Theatre case

One visit of a patient to an operating theatre to undergo one or more operative procedures.

Operating theatre

A room in a hospital on site containing one or two operating tables or other similar devices. An operating theatre accommodates one or two patients at a time during and only during the period in which, under the direct supervision of a medical or dental practitioner, the patient (s) can undergo operative treatment .... for the prevention, cure, relief or diagnosis of disease.

The following are <u>excluded</u> from this description:

a) Obstetric delivery room containing a delivery bed
b) Dental treatment room or surgery containing a dental chair
c) X-ray room, whether diagnostic or therapeutic
d) Room only used to carry out endoscopy

Scheduled session: during or outside

Theatre cases are classified by whether the visit to the operating theatre occurred "during" or "outside" a scheduled session. A theatre case is considered "during" if it was carried out during a period of time allocated to a scheduled operating theatre session and by a member of a consultant firm of the same specialty as that allocated to the session. Note that a scheduled operating theatre session may overrun.

A theatre case is "outside" a scheduled operating theatre session if it is not "during".

Operating theatre session type

A. Scheduled primarily for theatre cases planned in advance. Periods of theatre time allocated to a consultant, usually on a regular basis, in which the consultant or a member of the firm can perform operations, the majority of which have been arranged beforehand. The maximum duration of a scheduled session is a notional half-day.

B. Scheduled primarily for emergency theatre cases. Periods of time allocated to a consultant on a regular basis for patients whose visit to the operating theatre was not foreseen but takes place as a result of illness or complication requiring an urgent operation. The maximum duration of a session is a notional half-day.

C. Unscheduled. Periods of time allocated to one or more consultants, outside scheduled sessions allocated to a consultant and used by that consultant or one of the same specialty, for specific theatre cases, usually at short notice.

Theatre case: start time

The start of anaesthesia of the patient where this takes place either in the operating theatre or in the anaesthetic room, or start of the procedure(s) if no anaesthetic is given.

Theatre case: time out of theatre

The time a theatre case leaves the operating theatre.
(NB not the time of leaving the theatre suite).

Theatre case: routine or emergency

Routine theatre cases: patients for whom arrangements have been made in advance. These cases may have been admitted to hospital either electively or as emergencies.

Emergency theatre cases: patients whose visit to the operating theatre was not foreseen but takes place as a result of illness or a complication requiring an urgent operation. These cases may have been admitted to hospital either electively or as emergencies and the operation may take place during or outside either type of scheduled session.

* Definitions taken from the NHS Data Dictionary Version 1.1, Volume 2 (NHS Management Executive March 1994)

Appendix D

APPENDIX E

Table E1
Procedures performed between 18.01 and 21.00 hrs, Monday to Friday and Saturday or Sunday
(Grouped by specialty of the consultant surgeon heading the team)

Cardiothoracic

OPCS4 Codes	Description	Monday to Friday	Saturday or Sunday
E51	Diagnostic endoscopic examination of lower respiratory tract using rigid bronchoscope	2	0
E54	Excision of lung	1	0
E63	Diagnostic endoscopic examination of mediastinum	1	0
G15	Other therapeutic endoscopic operation on oesophagus	1	0
G18	Therapeutic endoscopic operation on oesophagus using rigid oesophagoscope	1	0
K40	Saphenous vein graft replacement of coronary artery	2	0
K43	Prosthetic replacement of coronary artery	5	0
K44	Other replacement of coronary artery	3	0
K49	Transluminal balloon angioplasty of coronary artery	1	0
S06	Excision of lesion of skin	1	0
S57	Debridement of skin	1	0
T03	Opening of chest	2	0
T05	Other operation on chest wall	1	0
T10	Therapeutic endoscopic operation on pleura	1	0
Unable to code		1	1

General surgery (including vascular surgery)

OPCS4 Codes	Description	Monday to Friday	Saturday or Sunday
A27	Extracranial extirpation of vagus nerve	1	0
A41	Drainage of subdural space	1	0
B32	Biopsy of breast	1	0
B33	Incision of breast	2	1
B37	Other operation on breast	1	0
E02	Plastic operation on nose	1	0
E42	Exteriorisation of trachea	0	1
F05 & F06	Repair of /operation on lip	1	1
F18	Excision of dental lesion of jaw	1	0
F26	Operation on tongue	1	0
F34	Excision of tonsil	4	1
F46	Incision of salivary gland	1	0
G03	Partial excision of oesophagus	1	0
G08	Artificial opening into oesophagus	1	0
G13	Other open operations on oesophagus	1	0
G15	Therapeutic fibreoptic endoscopic operations on oesophagus	3	0
G28	Partial excision of stomach	2	0
G35	Operation on ulcer of stomach	0	1
G40	Incision of pylorus	2	0
G43	Fibreoptic endoscopic extirpation of lesion of upper gastrointestinal tract	0	1
G44	Other fibreoptic therapeutic endoscopic operations on upper gastrointestinal tract	0	1
G45	Diagnostic fibreoptic endoscopic examination of upper gastrointestinal tract	15	0
G52	Operations on ulcer of duodenum	7	0
G53	Other open operations on duodenum	1	0
G58	Excision of jejunum	1	0
G61	Bypass of jejunum	1	0
G65	Diagnostic endoscopic examination of jejunum	0	1
G69	Excision of ileum	1	0

Appendix E (table E1, evening operations, 18.01 to 21.00 hrs)

General surgery (including vascular surgery) continued

Code	Description		
G71	Bypass of ileum	4	0
G72	Other connection of ileum	0	1
G74	Creation of artificial opening into ileum	2	0
G75	Attention to artificial opening into ileum	1	1
G76	Intraabdominal manipulation of ileum	1	0
G78	Other open operations on ileum	6	1
H01	Emergency excision of appendix	86	35
H02	Other excision of appendix	15	6
H03	Other operations on appendix	1	0
H07	Excision of right hemicolon	4	0
H08	Excision of transverse colon	2	1
H10	Excision of sigmoid colon	1	0
H11	Other excision of colon	4	1
H15	Exteriorisation of colon	3	0
H17	Intraabdominal manipulation of colon	0	1
H20	Endoscopic extirpation of lesion of colon	0	1
H21	Therapeutic endoscopic operations on colon	1	0
H22	Diagnostic endoscopic examination of colon	1	0
H25	Diagnostic endoscopic examination of lower bowel using fibreoptic sigmoidoscope	1	0
H28	Diagnostic endoscopic examination of sigmoid colon using rigid sigmoidoscope	3	0
H30	Other operations on colon	0	1
H33	Excision of rectum	18	1
H44	Manipulation of rectum	4	0
H46	Operations on rectum	1	0
H48	Excision of lesion of anus	1	0
H51	Excision of haemorrhoid	3	2
H52	Destruction of haemorrhoid	2	0
H53	Other operations on haemorrhoid	2	0
H54	Dilation of anal sphincter	4	0
H55	Other operations on perianal region	2	2
H56	Other operations on anus	1	0
H58	Drainage through perineal region	25	10
H59	Excision of pilonidal sinus	1	0
H60	Other operations on pilonial sinus	13	3
H62	Other operations on bowel	2	0
J01	Transplantation of liver	1	0
J05	Incision of liver	1	0
J18	Excision of gall bladder	5	1
J21	Incision of gall bladder	3	0
J31	Open introduction of prosthesis into bile duct	1	0
J40	Endoscopic retrograde placement of prosthesis in bile duct	0	1
J50	Percutaneous examination of bile duct	1	0
J55	Total excision of pancreas	1	-
J69	Total excision of spleen	2	0
L18	Emergency replacement of aneurysmal segment of aorta	3	1
L19	Other replacement of aneurysmal segment of aorta	1	0
L20	Other emergency bypass of segment of aorta	1	0
L25	Open operations on aorta	1	1
L38	Open operations on subclavian artery	2	1
L50	Emergency bypass of iliac artery	1	0
L53	Open operations on iliac artery	1	0
L58	Emergency bypass of femoral artery	1	0
L59	Other bypass of femoral artery	2	0
L62	Other open operations on femoral artery	5	0
L63	Transluminal operations on femoral artery	1	0
L67	Excision of other artery	2	0

General surgery (including vascular surgery) continued

Code	Description		
L68	Repair of other artery	1	0
L70	Other open operations on other artery	3	0
L74	Arteriovenous shunt	0	1
L85	Ligation of varicose vein of leg	6	0
L87	Other operations on varicose vein of leg	3	0
L90	Open removal of thrombus from vein	1	0
L91	Other vein related operations	8	0
M01	Transplantation of kidney	2	1
M42	Endoscopic extirpation of lesion of bladder	1	0
M65	Endoscopic resection of outlet of male bladder	1	0
N03	Operations on scrotum	1	0
N07	Extirpation of lesion of testis	1	0
N09	Other placement of testis in scrotum	1	0
N11	Operations on hydrocele sac	1	0
N13	Other operations on testis	3	0
N30	Operations on prepuce	5	0
Q11	Evacuation of contents of uterus	0	1
Q43	Partial excision of ovary	1	0
Q55	Examination of femal genital tract	0	1
S06	Excision of lesion of skin	8	1
S15	Biopsy of skin	1	0
S30	Operations on flap of skin to head or neck	1	0
S41	Suture of skin of head or neck	1	0
S42	Suture of skin of other site	2	2
S47	Opening of skin	28	10
S56	Exploration of other skin of head or neck	1	0
S57	Exploration of skin of other site	8	0
S70	Operations on nail	1	0
T05	Operations on chest wall	1	0
T12	Puncture of pleura	1	0
T20	Primary repair of inguinal hernia	7	1
T22	Primary repair of femoral hernia	6	2
T24	Repair of umbilical hernia	3	0
T25	Primary repair of incisional hernia	1	1
T27	Repair of other hernia of abdominal wall	1	1
T28	Other repair of anterior abdominal wall	1	0
T30	Opening of abdomen	16	4
T31	Other operations on anterior abdominal wall	3	1
T34	Open drainage of peritoneum	1	0
T41	Other open operations on peritoneum	9	2
T43	Diagnostic endoscopic examination of peritoneum	4	1
T87	Excision or biopsy of lymph node	2	0
T88	Drainage of lesion of lymph node	1	0
W19	Primary open reduction of fracture of bone and intramedullary fixation	1	0
W26	Other closed reduction of fracture of bone	2	1
W48	Other prosthetic replacement of head of femur	0	1
W90	Puncture of joint	1	0
X01	Replantation of upper limb	0	1
X09	Amputation of leg	10	4
X11	Amputation of toe	4	0
X12	Operations on amputation stump	1	0
Y11	Cauterisation of organ	0	1
Y22	Drainage of organ	6	0
Y29	Removal of foreign body from organ	1	0
Unable to code		9	0

Appendix E (table E1, evening operations, 18.01 to 21.00 hrs)

Gynaecology

OPCS4 Codes	Description	Monday to Friday	Saturday or Sunday
A52	Therapeutic epidural injection	0	1
M79	Operations on urethra	1	0
P03	Operations on Bartholin gland	5	0
P05	Excision of vulva	0	1
P09	Other operation on vulva	1	0
P24	Repair of vault of vagina	1	0
P26	Intro of supporting pessary into vagina	1	0
P29	Other operations on vagina	2	0
Q02	Destruction of lesion of cervix uteri	1	0
Q03	Biopsy of cervix uteri	1	0
Q07	Abdominal excision of uterus	3	0
Q10	Curettage of uterus	24	4
Q11	Other evacuation of contents of uterus	256	27
Q12	Intrauterine contraceptive device	1	0
Q20	Other operations on uterus	1	0
Q23	Unilateral excision of adnexa of uterus	8	1
Q24	Other excision of adnexa of uterus	4	1
Q25	Partial excision of fallopian tube	2	1
Q30	Other repair of fallopian tube	2	0
Q31	Incision of fallopian tube	3	0
Q32	Operations on fimbria	1	0
Q38	Therapeutic endoscopic operations on fallopian tube	1	0
Q43	Partial excision of ovary	6	1
Q49	Therapeutic endoscopic operations on ovary	2	1
Q55	Other examination of female genital tract	0	1
S47	Opening of skin	2	0
T20	Primary repair of inguinal hernia	0	1
T30	Opening of abdomen	3	0
T31	Other operations on anterior abdominal	1	0
T41	Other open operations on peritoneum	2	0
T42	Therapeutic endoscopic operations on peritoneum	1	0
T43	Diagnostic endoscopic examinations of peritoneum	23	0
Y22	Drainage of organ	0	1

Neurosurgery

OPCS4 Codes	Description	Monday to Friday	Saturday or Sunday
A08	Biopsy of lesion of tissue of brain	1	1
A10	Other operations on tissue of brain	1	0
A12	Creation of connection from ventricle of brain	8	2
A14	Other operations on connection from ventricle of brain	6	1
A16	Other open operations on ventricle of brain	1	0
A20	Other operations on ventricle of brain	2	1
A41	Drainage of subdural space	8	2
A53	Drainage of spinal canal	2	0
D28	EUA of ear	1	0
E42	Exteriorisation of trachea	2	0
L29	Reconstruction of carotid artery	1	0
L33	Operations on aneurysm of cerebral artery	1	0
S42	Suture of skin	1	0
V03	Opening of cranium	3	1

Appendix E (table E1, evening operations, 18.01 to 21.00 hrs)

Ophthalmology

OPCS4 Codes	Description	Monday to Friday	Saturday or Sunday
C15	Correction of deformity of eyelid	2	0
C17	Other repair of eyelid	2	0
C46	Plastic operations on cornea	2	0
C47	Closure of cornea	1	0
C54	Buckling operations for attachment of retina	1	0
C57	Other operations on sclera	0	1
C61	Other operations on trabecular meshwork of eye	1	0
C66	Extirpation of ciliary body	1	0
C71	Extracapsular extraction of lens	9	0
C75	Prosthesis of lens	3	0
C77	Other operation on lens	1	0
C79	Operations on vitreous body	5	0
C81	Photocoagulation of retina for detachment	3	2
C82	Destruction of lesion of retina	2	0
C84	Other operations on retina	1	0
C86	Other operations on eye	1	0

Orthopaedic and trauma (including spinal injuries and hand surgery)

OPCS4 Codes	Description	Monday to Friday	Saturday or Sunday
A65	Release of entrapment of peripheral nerve at wrist	1	0
E42	Exteriorisation of trachea	1	0
E51	Diagnostic endoscopic examination of lower respiratory tract using rigid bronchoscope	1	0
G45	Diagnostic fibreopic endoscopic examination of upper gastrointestinal tract	1	0
H58	Drainage through perineal region	1	0
J69	Total excision of spleen	1	0
L72	Arteriography	0	1
M45	Diagnostic endoscopic examination of bladder	3	0
S06	Excision of lesion of skin	1	0
S35	Split autograft of skin	0	1
S42	Suture of skin	6	4
S45	Removal of foreign body from skin	7	0
S47	Opening of skin	9	3
S56	Exploration of other skin of head or neck	1	0
S57	Exploration of other skin of other site	25	5
S70	Operation on nail	1	1
T54	Division of fascia	0	1
T62	Operation on bursa	1	0
T67	Primary repair of tendon	19	4
T69	Freeing of tendon	1	0
T70	Adjustment to length of tendon	1	0
T72	Operation on sheath of tendon	2	0
T79	Repair of muscle	1	0
T83	Other operation on muscle	0	2
V15	Reduction of fracture of mandible	1	0
V24	Decompression operation on thoracic spine	2	0
V25	Primary decompression operations on lumbar spine	2	0
V26	Revisional decompression operation on lumbar spine	1	0
V33	Primary excision of lumbar intervertebral disc	2	0
V46	Fixation of fracture of spine	1	0
V52	Other operation on intervertebral disc	1	0
W06	Total excision of coccyx	1	0
W08	Partial excision of bone	1	0

Appendix E (table E1, evening operations, 18.01 to 21.00 hrs)

Orthopaedic and trauma (including spinal injuries and hand surgery) continued

Code	Description		
W19.1	Primary open reduction of fracture of neck of femur and open fixation using pin and plate	27	9
W19.2	Primary open reduction of fracture of long bone and fixation using rigid nail	0	1
W19.3	Primary open reduction of fracture of long bone and fixation using flexible nail	1	1
W19.5	Primary open reduction of fragment of bone and fixation using screw	3	1
W19.6	Primary open reduction of fragment of bone and fixation using wire system	4	0
W19.8	Other specified	12	5
W19.9	Unspecified	21	5
W20	Primary open reduction of fracture of bone and extramedullary fixation	10	7
W21	Primary open reduction of intraarticular fracture of bone	0	1
W22	Other primary open reduction of fracture of bone	1	1
W24	Closed reduction of fracture of bone and internal fixation	3	2
W25	Closed reduction of fracture of bone and external fixation	2	1
W26	Other closed reduction of fracture of bone	68	44
W28	Other internal fixation of bone	38	6
W29	Skeletal traction of bone	1	1
W30	Other external fixation of bone	6	3
W33	Other open operations on bone	1	1
W37	Total prosthetic replacement of hip joint using cement	2	1
W38	Total prosthetic replacement of hip joint not using cement	0	1
W39	Other total prosthetic replacement of hip joint	1	0
W42	Total prosthetic replacement of knee joint	2	0
W46	Prosthetic replacement of head of femur using cement	2	1
W47	Prosthetic replacement of head of femur not using cement	4	3
W48	Other prosthetic replacement of head of femur	14	1
W51	Prosthetic replacement of head of humerus	1	0
W65	Primary open reduction of traumatic dislocation of joint	3	0
W66	Primary closed reduction of traumatic dislocation of joint	10	4
W67	Secondary reduction of traumatic dislocation of joint	1	0
W69	Open operations on synovial membrane of joint	1	0
W77	Stabilising operation on joint	1	0
W81	Other open operations on joint	7	3
W82	Therapeutic endoscopic operations on semilunar cartilage	2	0
W85	Therapeutic endoscopic operations on cavity of knee joint	3	1
W87	Diagnostic endoscopic examination of knee joint	4	0
W90	Puncture of joint	1	1
W91	Other manipulation of joint	24	8
W92	Examination of joint under image intensifier	1	1
X08	Amputation of hand	3	0
X09	Amputation of leg	0	1
X10	Amputation of foot	1	0
Y22	Drainage of organ	1	0
Y29	Removal of foreign body from organ	1	0
Y31	Exploration of organ	1	0
Unable to code		6	1

Oral/maxillofacial/dental

OPCS4 Codes	Description	Monday to Friday	Saturday or Sunday
F05	Repair of lip	1	0
F09	Surgical removal of tooth	6	1
F10	Simple extraction of tooth	3	0
F16	Other operations on tooth	1	0
F18	Excision of dental lesion of jaw	2	0
F40	Suture of mouth	0	1
S41	Suture of skin of head or neck	5	0
S42	Suture of skin, other site	1	0
S47	Opening of skin	1	0
S57	Debridement of skin	0	1
V08	Reduction of fracture of maxilla	1	0
V09	Reduction of fracture of other bone of face	5	1
V11	Fixation of bone of face	3	0
V15	Reduction of fracture of mandible	1	0
V17	Fixation of mandible	4	2
V20	Reconstruction of temporo-mandibular joint	1	0
W28	Removal of internal fixation from bone	1	0
Unable to code		0	1

Otorhinolaryngology

OPCS4 Codes	Description	Monday to Friday	Saturday or Sunday
D04	Drainage of external ear	0	1
D10	Exenteration of mastoid air cells	1	0
D15	Drainage of middle ear	0	1
E03	Operations on septum of nose	3	0
E04	Operations on turbinate of nose	2	0
E08	Other operations on internal nose	2	0
E14	Operations on frontal sinus	2	0
E27	Other operations on pharynx	0	1
E42	Exteriorisation of trachea	1	0
E49/E51	Diagnostic fibreoptic endoscopic examination of lower respiratory tract	2	1
F34/F36	Excision/other operations of tonsil	5	0
G15	Therapeutic fibreoptic endoscopic operation on oesophagus	0	1
S41/S47	Suture of skin	1	1
T03	Opening of chest	1	0

Paediatric

OPCS4 Codes	Description	Monday to Friday	Saturday or Sunday
A12	Creation of connection from ventricle of brain	1	1
E51	Diagnostic endoscopic examination of lower respiratory tract using rigid bronchoscope	1	0
G16/G19	Diagnostic fibreoptic endoscopic examination of oesophagus	2	0
G23	Repair of diaphragmatic hernia	1	0
G45	Diagnostic fibreoptic endoscopic examination of upper gastrointestinal tract	1	0
G69	Excision of ileum	1	0
G75	Attention to artificial opening into ileum	1	0
H01	Emergency excision of appendix	5	1
H02	Other excision of appendix	1	0
L91	Insertion of central venous catheter	2	0
M79	Dilation of urethra	1	0

Appendix E (table E1, evening operations, 18.01 to 21.00 hrs)

Paediatric continued

		Mon–Fri	Sat/Sun
N03	Exploration of scrotum	2	0
N13	Fixation of testis	1	0
S06	Excision of lesion, head or neck	1	0
S47	Opening of skin	3	0
S57	Debridement/toilet of skin	2	0

Plastic

OPCS4 Codes	Description	Monday to Friday	Saturday or Sunday
A64	Repair of peripheral nerve	3	1
A73	Other operation on peripheral nerve	0	1
B31	Plastic operation on breast	1	0
D01	Excision of external ear	1	0
D06	Repair of external ear	0	1
E03	Operations on septum of nose	1	0
E09	Operations on external nose	0	1
F05	Repair of lip	3	1
F24	Incision of tongue	1	0
S02	Plastic excision of skin of abdominal wall	2	0
S06	Excision of lesion of skin	3	0
S35	Split autograft of skin	2	0
S37	Other graft of skin	1	0
S41	Suture of skin of head or neck	2	0
S42	Suture of skin of other site	5	6
S44	Removal of inorganic substance from skin	1	0
S45	Removal of other substance from skin	2	0
S47	Opening of skin	1	0
S56	Exploration of other skin of head or neck	3	1
S57	Exploration of other skin of other site	14	3
S66	Operations on nail bed	1	0
T52	Revision of palmar fasciectomy	2	0
T67	Primary repair of tendon	12	4
T72	Operation on sheath of tendon	1	0
T77	Excision of muscle	0	1
T79	Repair of muscle	2	0
W16	Division of bone	1	0
W19	Primary open reduction of fracture of bone and intramedullary fixation	3	0
W20	Primary open reduction of fracture of bone and extramedullary fixation	1	0
W24	Closed reduction of fracture of bone and internal fixation	0	1
W26	Other closed reduction of fracture of bone	2	1
W28	Other internal fixation of bone	3	3
W81	Exploration of joint	1	2
X08	Amputation of hand	2	1
X09	Amputation of leg	1	0
Y22	Drainage of organ	1	0
Unable to code		2	0

Appendix E (table E1, evening operations, 18.01 to 21.00 hrs)

Urology

OPCS4 Codes	Description	Monday to Friday	Saturday or Sunday
L91	Removal of Portacath	1	0
M01	Transplantation of kidney	2	1
M29	Endoscopic insertion of tubal prosthesis into ureter	2	0
M30	Endoscopic retrograde pyelography	3	0
M37	Repair of rupture of bladder	0	1
M42	Endoscopic extirpation of lesion of bladder	3	0
M43	Endoscopic overdistension of bladder	1	0
M44	Endoscopic removal of blood clot from bladder	1	0
M45	Diagnostic endoscopic examination of bladder	4	0
M47	Urethral irrigation of bladder	1	0
M65	Endoscopic resection of prostate	4	0
N03	Other operations on scrotum	1	0
N06	Other excision of testis	1	0
N13	Other operations on testis	1	1
N17	Excision of vas deferens	1	0
N28	Plastic operations on penis	1	0
N30	Operations on prepuce	3	0
S42	Suture of skin	0	1
T27	Repair of hernia of abdominal wall	1	0
T28	Other repair of anterior abdominal wall	1	0
T30	Opening of abdomen	1	0
T34	Open drainage of peritoneum	1	0
T88	Drainage of lesion of lymph node	1	0
Y22	Drainage of organ	2	0

Appendix E (table E1, evening operations, 18.01 to 21.00 hrs)

Table E2

Procedures performed between 21.01 hrs to 24.00 hrs, Monday to Friday and Saturday or Sunday
(Grouped by specialty of the consultant surgeon heading the team)

Cardiothoracic

OPCS4 Codes	Description	Monday to Friday	Saturday or Sunday
E53	Transplantation of lung	1	0
K02	Transplantation of heart	4	1
K26	Plastic repair of aortic valve	2	0
K40	Saphenous vein graft replacement of coronary artery	0	1
K43	Prosthetic replacement of coronary artery	1	0
L70	Ligation of artery	0	1
T03	Opening of chest	0	1
T12	Puncture of pleura	1	0
Y32	Re-exploration of organ and surgical arrest of postop bleeding	1	0
Unable to code		1	0

General surgery (including vascular surgery)

OPCS4 Codes	Description	Monday to Friday	Saturday or Sunday
A27	Extracranial extirpation of vagus nerve	2	1
B33	Incision of breast	5	1
D04	Drainage of external ear	1	1
E42	Exteriorisation of trachea	1	0
F05/F06	Repair of/operation on lip	1	0
F26	Operation on tongue	0	1
F34	Excision of tonsil	0	1
F38	Excision of mouth lesion	1	0
G21	Intubation of oesophagus	0	1
G34	Artificial opening into stomach	1	0
G35	Operation on ulcer of stomach	2	0
G45	Diagnostic fibreoptic endoscopic examination of upper gastrointestinal tract	3	1
G52	Operations on ulcer of duodenum	7	4
G61	Bypass of jejunum	1	0
G63	Closure of perforation of jejunum	1	0
G69	Excision of ileum	2	2
G70	Excision of lesion of ileum	1	0
G71	Bypass of ileum	1	1
G74	Creation of artificial opening into ileum	0	1
G76	Intraabdominal manipulation of ileum	1	0
G78	Other open operations on ileum	6	1
H01	Emergency excision of appendix	105	23
H02	Other excision of appendix	25	3
H03	Other operations on appendix	1	1
H05	Total colectomy and ileostomy	1	0
H06	Extended excision of right hemicolon	3	0
H07	Excision of right hemicolon	6	0
H10	Excision of sigmoid colon	4	0
H15	Exteriorisation of colon	2	3
H28	Diagnostic endoscopic examination of sigmoid colon using rigid sigmoidoscope	2	0
H33	Excision of rectum	8	1
H44	Manipulation of rectum	1	0
H51	Excision of haemorrhoid	3	2

General surgery (including vascular surgery) continued

Code	Operation		
H53	Other operations on haemorrhoid	1	0
H54	Dilation of anal sphincter	2	0
H55	Other operations on perianal region	1	0
H56	Other operations on anus	2	0
H58	Drainage through perineal region	19	8
H59	Excision of pilonidal sinus	2	1
H60	Other operations on pilonidal sinus	11	4
J02	Partial excision of liver	0	1
J14	Biopsy of liver	1	0
J32	Repair of bile duct	1	0
J50	Percutaneous examination of bile duct	0	1
J61	Open drainage of lesion of pancreas	0	1
L18	Emergency replacement of aneurysmal segment of aorta	2	0
L25	Open operations on aorta	3	0
L30	Open embolectomy of carotid artery	1	0
L46	Operation on aneurysm of visceral branch of abdominal aorta	1	0
L51	Other bypass of iliac artery	1	0
L58	Emergency bypass of femoral artery	1	0
L62	Other open operations on femoral artery	3	2
L70	Other open operations on other artery	0	2
L91	Other vein related operations	5	0
M47	Urethral cauterisation of bladder	1	0
M65	Endoscopic resection of outlet of male bladder	1	0
N03	Operations on scrotum	4	0
N07	Extirpation of lesion of testis	1	0
N13	Other operations on testis	8	0
N20	Other operation on spermatic cord	1	0
N30	Operations on prepuce	0	1
P03	Operation on Bartholin gland	1	0
P31	Operation on pouch of Douglas	0	1
Q07	Abdominal excision of uterus	1	0
Q10	Curettage of uterus	1	0
Q24	Salpingo-oophorectomy	0	1
Q30	Salpingostomy	1	0
Q43	Partial excision of ovary	1	0
S41	Suture of skin of head or neck	0	1
S42	Suture of skin of other site	3	2
S47	Opening of skin	23	3
S57	Exploration of skin of other site	5	2
S60	Refashioning of scar	1	0
T19	Unilateral herniotomy	1	0
T20/T21	Primary repair of inguinal hernia	12	5
T22	Primary repair of femoral hernia	4	3
T24	Repair of umbilical hernia	4	2
T25	Primary repair of incisional hernia	2	1
T27	Repair of other hernia of abdominal wall	1	1
T28	Other repair of anterior abdominal wall	1	0
T29	Excision of urachus	0	1
T30	Opening of abdomen	10	4
T31	Other operations on anterior abdominal wall	0	1
T34	Open drainage of peritoneum	1	0
T36	Operation on omentum	1	0
T38	Operation on mesentery of colon	1	0
T41	Other open operations on peritoneum	8	1
T42	Endoscopic division of adhesions of peritoneum	1	0
T43	Diagnostic endoscopic examination of peritoneum	1	0
T54	Division of fascia	1	0
T87	Excision or biopsy of lymph node	1	0

Appendix E (table E2, evening operations, 21.01 to 24.00 hrs)

General surgery (including vascular surgery) continued

		Monday to Friday	Saturday or Sunday
W26	Other closed reduction of fracture of bone	4	1
W90	Puncture of joint	1	1
X09	Amputation of leg	5	0
X11	Amputation of toe	2	0
Y18	Freeing of adhesions of organ	1	0
Y22	Drainage of organ	2	2
Y29	Removal of foreign body from organ	1	1
Y32	Re-exploration of organ	1	0
Unable to code		4	2

Gynaecology

OPCS4 Codes	Description	Monday to Friday	Saturday or Sunday
B33	Incision of breast	2	0
G69	Excision of ileum	1	0
L70	Ligation of artery	1	0
M75	Open biopsy of lesion of urethra	1	0
P03	Operations on Bartholin gland	6	0
P09	Other operation on vulva	4	0
P23	Anterior and posterior colporrhaphy	1	0
P25	Suture of vagina	1	0
P31	Operations on pouch of Douglas	1	0
Q02	Destruction of lesion of cervix uteri	3	0
Q10	Curettage of uterus	13	0
Q11	Other evacuation of contents of uterus	148	16
Q23	Unilateral excision of adnexa of uterus	10	1
Q24	Other excision of adnexa of uterus	2	1
Q25	Partial excision of fallopian tube	2	1
Q30	Other repair of fallopian tube	1	0
Q31	Incision of fallopian tube	3	0
Q43	Partial excision of ovary	2	0
Q49	Therapeutic endoscopic operations on ovary	3	0
S47	Opening of skin	1	1
T28	Suture of anterior abdominal wall	1	0
T30	Opening of abdomen	4	0
T43	Diagnostic endoscopic examinations of peritoneum	10	0
Y32	Re-exploration of organ	1	0

Neurosurgery

OPCS4 Codes	Description	Monday to Friday	Saturday or Sunday
A05	Drainage of abscess of tissue of brain	3	0
A07	Other open operation on tissue of brain	0	1
A08	Biopsy of lesion of tissue of brain	1	0
A12	Creation of connection from ventricle of brain	2	4
A14	Other operations on connection from ventricle of brain	5	0
A20	Other operations on ventricle of brain	4	0
A40	Drainage of extradural space	3	1
A41	Drainage of subdural space	7	0
L33	Operations on aneurysm of cerebral artery	1	0
V03	Opening of cranium	4	0
V05	Elevation of depressed fracture of cranium	0	1
V33	Primary excision of lumbar intervertebral disc	1	0
Unable to code		1	1

Appendix E (table E2, evening operations, 21.01 to 24.00 hrs)

Ophthalmology

OPCS4 Codes	Description	Monday to Friday	Saturday or Sunday
C10	Operation on eyebrow	0	1
C54	Buckling operations for attachment of retina	1	0
C79	Operations on vitreous body	1	0
C86	Other operations on eye	1	0

Orthopaedic and trauma (including spinal injuries and hand surgery)

OPCS4 Codes	Description	Monday to Friday	Saturday or Sunday
A62	Microsurgical repair of peripheral nerve	2	0
A64	Other repair of peripheral nerve	0	1
S06	Excision of lesion of skin	2	0
S24	Local flap of skin and muscle	1	0
S42	Suture of skin	3	3
S45	Removal of foreign body from skin	4	1
S47	Opening of skin	8	1
S56/S57	Exploration of skin	11	6
T30	Opening of abdomen	1	0
T54	Division of fascia	0	1
T62	Operation on bursa	1	0
T67	Primary repair of tendon	8	2
T72	Operation on sheath of tendon	2	0
T79	Repair of muscle	1	0
T83	Other operation on muscle	1	0
T96	Other operation on soft tissue	0	1
W08	Partial excision of bone	2	0
W19.1	Primary open reduction of fracture of neck of femur and open fixation using pin and plate	5	2
W19.5	Primary open reduction of fragment of bone and fixation using screw	1	0
W19.6	Primary open reduction of fragment of bone and fixation using wire system	2	0
W19.8	Other specified	10	1
W19.9	Unspecified	4	5
W20	Primary open reduction of fracture of bone and extramedullary fixation	6	1
W22	Other primary open reduction of fracture of bone	1	0
W24	Closed reduction of fracture of bone and internal fixation	2	0
W25	Closed reduction of fracture of bone and external fixation	4	0
W26	Other closed reduction of fracture of bone	82	41
W28	Other internal fixation of bone	9	7
W29	Skeletal traction of bone	1	0
W30	Other external fixation of bone	3	1
W33	Other open operations on bone	1	2
W39	Other total prosthetic replacement of hip joint	2	1
W46	Prosthetic replacement of head of femur using cement	1	1
W47	Prosthetic replacement of head of femur not using cement	0	1
W48	Other prosthetic replacement of head of femur	3	2
W51	Prosthetic replacement of head of humerus	1	0
W60	Fusion of joint and extraarticular bone graft	1	0
W65	Primary open reduction of traumatic dislocation of joint	2	0
W66	Primary closed reduction of traumatic dislocation of joint	7	5
W68	Primary reduction of injury to growth plate	1	0
W75	Other open repair of ligament	0	1
W77	Stabilising operation on joint	1	0
W81	Other open operations on joint	4	2
W85	Therapeutic endoscopic operations on cavity of knee joint	5	4
W87	Diagnostic endoscopic examination of knee joint	1	0
W90	Puncture of joint	3	0

Appendix E (table E2, evening operations, 21.01 to 24.00 hrs)

Orthopaedic and trauma (including spinal injuries and hand surgery) continued

W91	Other manipulation of joint	27	11
W92	Examination of joint under image intensifier	1	1
X08	Amputation of hand	2	0
Unable to code		6	1

Oral/maxillofacial/dental

OPCS4 Codes	Description	Monday to Friday	Saturday or Sunday
E09	Operations on external nose	1	1
F05	Repair of lip	2	0
F10	Simple extraction of tooth	1	0
F16	Other operations on tooth	3	0
F46	Incision of salivary gland	1	0
S41	Suture of skin of head or neck	4	2
S42	Suture of skin, other site	2	0
S47	Opening of skin	1	0
S56	Debridement of skin of head or neck	0	2
V09	Reduction of fracture of other bone of face	2	1
V14	Excision of mandible	0	1
V15	Reduction of fracture of mandible	2	1
V17	Fixation of mandible	2	1
W28	Removal of internal fixation from bone	1	0

Otorhinolaryngology

OPCS4 Codes	Description	Monday to Friday	Saturday or Sunday
D10	Exenteration of mastoid air cells	1	0
E03	Operations on septum of nose	2	0
E04	Operations on turbinate of nose	1	0
E06	Packing of cavity of nose	0	1
E20	Operation on adenoid	2	0
E25	Pharyngoscopy	1	0
E42	Exteriorisation of trachea	1	0
E51	Diagnostic fibreoptic endoscopic examination of lower respiratory tract	1	0
F34	Excision of tonsil	1	0
G15	Therapeutic fibreoptic endoscopic operation on oesophagus	3	1
E35	Endoscopic removal of foreign body from larynx	1	0
E36	Diagnostic endoscopic examination of larynx	1	1
G18	Endoscopic removal of foreign body from oesophagus	4	1
G44	Fibreoptic endoscopic removal of foreign body from upper gastrointestinal tract	1	0
S56	Exploration of skin	1	0

Paediatric

OPCS4 Codes	Description	Monday to Friday	Saturday or Sunday
F34	Excision of tonsil	2	0
G19	Diagnostic fibreoptic endoscopic examination of oesophagus	1	0
G76	Attention to artificial opening into ileum	2	0
H01	Emergency excision of appendix	2	1
H02	Other excision of appendix	2	1
H60	Drainage of pilonidal sinus	1	0
N03	Exploration of scrotum	0	1
N13	Fixation of testis	1	0
S41	Suture of skin of head or neck	1	0
S47	Opening of skin	2	1

Plastic

OPCS4 Codes	Description	Monday to Friday	Saturday or Sunday
A62	Microsurgical repair of peripheral nerve	2	0
A64	Repair of peripheral nerve	4	1
A73	Other operation on peripheral nerve	0	1
D01	Excision of external ear	0	1
D06	Repair of external ear	1	2
E05	Cauterisation of internal nose	1	0
F05	Repair of lip	1	4
S35	Split autograft of skin	2	1
S36	Other autograft of skin	0	1
S41	Suture of skin of head or neck	1	1
S42	Suture of skin of other site	4	2
S44	Removal of inorganic substance from skin	4	1
S47	Opening of skin	3	0
S56	Exploration of other skin of head or neck	2	0
S57	Exploration of other skin of other site	11	3
T51	Excision of fascia of abdomen	1	0
T67	Primary repair of tendon	8	0
T72	Operation on sheath of tendon	1	0
W19	Primary open reduction of fracture of bone and intramedullary fixation	1	0
W28	Other internal fixation of bone	1	1
W75	Open repair of ligament	1	0
X01	Replantation of upper limb	1	0
Unable to code		2	1

Urology

OPCS4 Codes	Description	Monday to Friday	Saturday or Sunday
E42	Exteriorisation of trachea	1	0
H15	Loop colostomy	1	0
H60	Drainage of pilonidal sinus	1	0
L91	Removal of Portacath	0	1
M29	Endoscopic insertion of tubal prosthesis into ureter	2	0
M42	Endoscopic extirpation of lesion of bladder	1	0
N03	Other operations on scrotum	2	0
N07	Extirpation of lesion of testis	1	0
N11	Excision of hydrocele sac	1	0
N13	Other operations on testis	1	1
N32	Operation on penis	0	1
S42	Suture of skin	1	0
T30	Opening of abdomen	0	1
Y22	Drainage of organ	1	0
Unable to code		2	0

Appendix E (table E2, evening operations, 21.01 to 24.00 hrs)

Table E3
Procedures performed between 00.01 hrs and 07.59 hrs, Monday to Friday and Saturday or Sunday
(Grouped by specialty of the consultant surgeon heading the team)

Cardiothoracic

OPCS4 Codes	Description	Monday to Friday	Saturday or Sunday
E53	Transplantation of lung	1	0
K01	Transplantation of heart and lung	1	0
K02	Other transplantation of heart	2	0
K04	Correction of tetralogy of Fallot	0	1
K22	Other operation on wall of atrium	1	0
K44	Other replacement of coronary artery	0	1
K23/E54	Other operation of wall of heart, and excision of lung	1	0
L18	Emergency replacement of aneurysmal segment of aorta	1	0
T03	Opening of chest	3	1
T12	Puncture of pleura	1	0

General surgery (including vascular surgery)

OPCS4 Codes	Description	Monday to Friday	Saturday or Sunday
A27	Extracranial extirpation of vagus nerve and incision of pylorus	0	1
B33	Incision of breast	2	2
E41	Tracheostomy	1	0
G28	Partial excision of stomach	1	1
G33	Other connection of stomach to jejunum	1	0
G35	Operation on ulcer of stomach	2	0
G36	Other repair of stomach	1	0
G45	Diagnostic fibreoptic endoscopic examination of upper gastrointestinal tract	2	0
G51	Bypass of duodenum	1	0
G52	Operations on ulcer of duodenum	5	2
G74	Creation of artificial opening into ileum	1	0
G78	Other open operations on ileum	2	2
H01	Emergency excision of appendix	56	14
H02	Other excision of appendix	13	4
H05	Total excision of colon	1	6
H07/H15	Other excision of right hemicolon/exteriorisation of colon	2	6
H10	Excision of sigmoid colon	2	
H11	Other excision of colon	1	1
H15	Other exteriorisation of colon	0	
H28	Diagnostic endoscopic examination of sigmoid colon using rigid sigmoidoscope	2	
H33	Excision of rectum	2	
H48	Excision of lesion of anus	1	
H58	Drainage through perineal region	6	
H60	Other operations on pilonidal sinus	8	
H62	Other operations on bowel	0	
J69	Total excision of spleen	1	
L18	Emergency replacement of aneurysmal segment of aorta	1	
L23	Plastic repair of aorta	1	
L25	Other open operations on aorta	3	
L38	Other open operations on subclavian artery	2	
L59	Other bypass of femoral artery	1	
L62	Other open operations on femoral artery	2	
L70	Other open operations on other artery	3	
L91	Other vein related operations	0	

General surgery (including vascular surgery) continued

Code	Description	Monday to Friday	Saturday or Sunday
M01	Transplantation of kidney	1	0
M02	Total excision of kidney	1	0
M08	Other open operations on kidney	1	0
M70	Other open operations on outlet of male bladder	1	0
N01	Extirpation of scrotum	0	1
N03	Other operation on scrotum	1	0
N06	Other excision of testis	1	0
N07	Extirpation of lesion of testes	0	1
N08	Bilateral placement of testes in scrotum	0	1
N09	Other placement of testis in scrotum	1	0
N13	Other operations on testis	2	2
N15	Operation on epididymis	1	0
N30	Operations on prepuce	2	1
S06	Other excision of lesion of skin	1	1
S42	Suture of skin	0	1
S44	Removal of inorganic substance from skin of back	1	0
S47	Opening of skin	11	3
S57	Exploration of other skin	3	1
T03/T05	Opening of chest/operation on chest wall	0	2
T19	Simple excision of inguinal hernia sac	0	1
T20	Primary repair of inguinal hernia	8	0
T21	Repair of recurrent inguinal hernia	1	0
T22	Primary repair of femoral hernia	5	0
T24	Repair of umbilical hernia	4	0
T26	Repair of recurrent incisional hernia	0	1
T28	Other repair of anterior abdominal wall	0	1
T30	Opening of abdomen	9	6
T31	Other operations on anterior abdominal wall	1	0
T34	Open drainage of peritoneum	2	2
T39	Operations on posterior peritoneum	1	0
T41	Other open operations on peritoneum	1	0
X09	Amputation of leg	1	0
X11	Amputation of toe	2	0
Unable to code		2	2

Gynaecology

OPCS4 Codes	Description	Monday to Friday	Saturday or Sunday
P03	Operations on Bartholin gland	4	1
P09	Other operation on vulva	2	1
P25	Other repair of vagina	1	1
P29	Operation on vagina	1	0
Q05	Other operation on cervix uteri	0	1
Q09	Other open operation on uterus	1	0
Q10	Curettage of uterus	5	0
Q11	Other evacuation of contents of uterus	41	14
Q18	Diagnostic endoscopic examination of uterus	1	0
Q23	Unilateral excision of adnexa of uterus	8	0
Q24	Other excision of adnexa of uterus	2	0
Q25	Partial excision of fallopian tube	3	1
Q31	Incision of fallopian tube	1	1
Q50	Diagnostic endoscopic examination of ovary	0	1
T43	Diagnostic endoscopic examination of peritoneum	7	1
Y22	Drainage of organ	1	0
Unable to code		0	1

Neurosurgery

OPCS4 Codes	Description	Monday to Friday	Saturday Sunday
A14	Open operations on connection from ventricle of brain	2	
A16	Other open operation on ventricle of brain	0	
A20	Other operations on ventricle of brain	3	
A39	Repair of dura	2	
A40	Drainage of extradural space	0	
A41	Drainage of subdural space	2	
V05	Operations on cranium	2	
V09	Reduction of fracture of bone of face	1	
V33	Primary excision of lumbar intervertebral disc	0	

Ophthalmology

OPCS4 Codes	Description	Monday to Friday	Saturday Sunday
C57	Repair of sclera	0	
C86	Removal of foreign body from eye	1	

Oral/maxillofacial/dental

OPCS4 Codes	Description	Monday to Friday	Saturday Sunday
F09	Surgical removal of tooth	1	
S41/S56	Suture of/exploration of skin of head or neck	1	
V17	Fixation of mandible	1	

Orthopaedic and trauma (including spinal injuries and hand surgery)

OPCS4 Codes	Description	Monday to Friday	Saturday Sunday
S42	Suture of skin	2	
S47	Opening of skin	1	
S56	Exploration of skin of head or neck	1	
S57	Debridement of skin	1	
T67	Primary repair of tendon	0	
V22	Primary anterior decompression of cervical spinal cord and fusion of joint of cervical spine	1	
W19	Primary open reduction of fracture of bone and intramedullary fixation	8	
W20	Primary open reduction of fracture of bone and extramedullary fixation	2	
W22	Other primary open reduction of fracture of bone	0	
W25	Closed reduction of fracture of bone and external fixation		
W26	Other closed reduction of fracture of bone	15	
W28	Other internal fixation of bone	2	
W30	Other external fixation of bone	1	
W33	Other open operations on bone	1	
W45	Total prosthetic replacement of joint	1	
W48	Other prosthetic replacement of head of femur	0	
W66	Primary closed reduction of traumatic dislocation of joint	5	
W77	Stabilising operations on joint	1	
W81	Other open operations on joint	4	
W90/W85	Puncture of joint/endoscopic operation on cavity of knee joint	1	
W91	Other manipulation of joint	6	
W92	Other operations on joint	1	
Unable to code		0	

Appendix E (table E3, night-time operations)

Otorhinolaryngology

OPCS4 Codes	Description	Monday to Friday	Saturday or Sunday
D14	Repair of eardrum	1	0
E03	Operation on septum of nose	1	0
E09	Operation on external nose	1	0
E27	Other operation on pharynx	0	1
E36/ E51	Diagnostic endoscopic examination of larynx, and lower respiratory tract	0	1
E42	Exteriorisation of trachea	0	1
F36	Operation on tonsil	1	4
G18	Therapeutic endoscopic operations on oesophagus using rigid oesophagoscope	1	1

Paediatric

OPCS4 Codes	Description	Monday to Friday	Saturday or Sunday
H17	Intraabdominal manipulation of colon	1	0
M47	Urethral catheterisation of bladder	1	0
N08	Bilateral placement of testes in scrotum	1	0
S47	Opening of skin	1	1
T30	Opening of abdomen	1	0
T96	Operation on soft tissue	1	0

Plastic

OPCS4 Codes	Description	Monday to Friday	Saturday or Sunday
F05	Repair of lip	4	0
S27	Local flap of skin	1	0
S35	Split autograft of skin (and repair of ulnar nerve)	0	1
S36	Other autograft of skin	1	0
S41	Suture of skin of head or neck	1	1
S42	Suture of skin of other site	2	0
S57	Exploration of skin of other site	0	2
S66	Operation on nail bed	1	0
T67	Primary repair of tendon	1	1
T79	Repair of muscle	1	0
V09	Reduction of fracture of bone of face	1	0

Urology

OPCS4 Codes	Description	Monday to Friday	Saturday or Sunday
L25	Operation on aneurysm of aorta	1	0
M21	Ileal replacement of ureter	1	0
M44	Therapeutic endoscopic operation on bladder	1	0
N07	Extirpation of lesion of testis	1	0
N13	Other operations on testis	3	0
S47	Opening of skin	0	1

APPENDIX F

All deaths reported by local reporters
1 April 1995 to 31 March 1996

Anglia & Oxford	1672
North Thames	2081
North West	2736
Northern & Yorkshire	3110
South & West	2508
South Thames	2166
Trent	2397
West Midlands	1595
Wales	840
Northern Ireland	469
Defence Medical Services	7
Guernsey	33
Jersey	26
Independent sector	201
Total	**19841**